Shared Care for Diabetes

Wendy Gatling FRCP

Consultant Physician, Poole Hospital NHS Trust, Poole, UK

Ron Hill FRCP

Consultant Physician, Poole Hospital NHS Trust, Poole, UK

Michael Kirby MRCP

Family Practitioner, The Surgery, Nevells Road, Letchworth, UK

Foreword by

Harry Keen FRCP

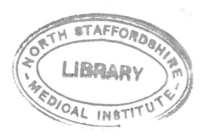

I S I S
MEDICAL
M E D I A

Oxford

© 1997 Isis Medical Media Ltd
58 St Aldates
Oxford OX1 1ST, UK

First published 1997

British Library Cataloguing in Publication Data
A catalogue record for this title is available from the British Library

ISBN 1 899066 25 X

Library of Congress
Cataloguing-in-Publication Data

Gatling, Wendy
Shared Care for Diabetes
Wendy Gatling, Ron Hill, Mike Kirby

Always refer to the manufacturer's Prescribing Information before prescribing
drugs cited in this book.

Typeset by
Creative Associates, 115 Magdalen Road, Oxford OX4 1RS, UK

Printed and bound by
Dah Hua Printing Press Co. Ltd., Hong Kong

Distributed by
Oxford University Press, Saxon Way West,
Corby, Northamptonshire NN18 9ES, UK

Contents

Foreword

The understanding and care of diabetes is a continuously evolving scene. It has advanced strikingly since I commenced my diabetic tutelage with Dr R D Lawrence almost 50 years ago and the pace shows no sign of slackening. Doctors Gatling, Hill and Kirby are to be congratulated for having portrayed the state of the diabetes art at the end of the millenium so effectively. They have shown notable success in getting the facts down on paper.

Much that they describe has lasting qualities. Indeed, the title, *Shared Care for Diabetes*, is an indication of a philosophy which has become central to the provision of comprehensive and effective care for diabetes as well as for many other medical conditions of long duration. The quality of care — and the quality of existence for the person with diabetes — depend critically upon the activities of many different people with many different skills, ideally working together to achieve agreed objectives. The authors rank 'co-operation' and 'integration' as two essential components of a sound and effective system of care. These are difficult enough to achieve and sustain, but even more so when the greatly differing needs of individual people with diabetes are considered. 'Flexibility' must be a third essential.

The contribution of each member of the therapeutic team receives consideration in the book. Based upon the particular circumstances of the operation of the National Health Service in the UK, for example in considering the relationships between primary care and hospital-based specialist services, the messages that emerge are actually very general and apply to most advanced and complex medical structures in industrialized countries. Central importance is rightly given to the role in the 'therapeutic partnership' of the person with diabetes and the desirability of 'patient empowerment' is considered in the light of an all too natural patient reluctance to accept it on occasions. The value of medical audit — looking at what one is doing and improving it — gets useful consideration.

Above all, the book contains much up-to-date, practical, clinical advice on the day-to-day treatment of diabetes and the management and prevention of diabetic emergencies. It is reader-friendly and a suitable diabetes *vade mecum* for the non-specialist and the enquiring patient and carer. In my opinion, its setting firmly within the framework of the Saint Vincent Declaration is to be greatly commended. In translating the ambitious but achievable goals of the Declaration into the daily business of diabetes care, the book makes a very substantial contribution to the improvement of the life and health of people with diabetes to whom, by whom and for whom the Declaration was made.

Professor Harry Keen MD FRCP
Vice President and late Chairman, British Diabetic Association
Honorary President, International Diabetes Federation
Emeritus Professor of Human Metabolism, Guy's Campus, UMDS
Consultant Emeritus, Guy's and St Thomas's Hospital, London, UK

Preface

The chronic nature of diabetes and the diversity of its long-term complications means that medical care of any diabetic patient is a long-term process involving a broad spectrum of different professional skills. Successful integration of these many aspects of care and a coordinated approach are vital for the provision of a high standard of care for all diabetic patients.

This book is intended as a guide for all health care professionals involved in the care of people with diabetes. Although the NHS system in the UK has provided a natural focus for the book, the basic principles of shared care are applicable to other health care systems worldwide. In this essentially practical guide to shared diabetes care, references are kept to a minimum, but ideas for further reading are included.

The authors would like to acknowledge the contributions of members of the diabetes team at Poole Hospital NHS Trust; Carolyn Smyth, dietitian, for her work on dietary aspects; Pam Hindley and Diane Clark, diabetes specialist nurses, for their contributions on education and home monitoring; Debbie Sharman and her team of podiatrists, particularly Debbie O'Halloran, who devised the foot assessment protocols; Joe Begley for his comments on the lipid sections, and Martin Crick for his advice on the retinopathy chapter.

Finally, we are particularly grateful to Carole Start, our medical editor, whose skill has been invaluable in the coordination of our individual contributions and our varying writing styles. Her insight and personal experience as a diabetic patient has helped to emphasize the importance of a patient-centred approach.

Wendy Gatling
Ron D. Hill
Michael G. Kirby

Chapter 1

Diabetes in profile

This introductory chapter briefly outlines those aspects of diabetes mellitus pertinent to shared care between the primary and secondary health care sectors. Further details can be found in later chapters and in the suggested further reading and references. This introduction concentrates on definition and classification of diabetes, its aetiology, pathology and epidemiology. Finally, the goals of treatment in the context of recent studies and in the light of the St Vincent Declaration are reviewed.

Defining diabetes

Diabetes mellitus is not a single disease entity but a group of diseases with common features, of which abnormal blood glucose homoeostasis and chronic hyperglycaemia are the basic clinical attributes. Its diagnosis (Chapter 2) is not problematic; blood glucose levels diagnostic of diabetes have been clearly defined by the WHO.

The importance of these values lies in their prognostic significance. Patients with diabetes carry in the long term a high risk of developing microvascular complications that are peculiar to diabetes. In addition, people with diabetes have a greater chance of developing more widespread macrovascular disease at a younger age than the remainder of the population.

Blood glucose homoeostasis

In non-diabetic people, the concentration of glucose in the blood is maintained within a narrow range, usually between 4 mmol/l and 7 mmol/l. This tight control is achieved by a delicately balanced response to factors tending to raise or lower blood glucose (Figure 1.1).

Insulin plays a pivotal role in these homoeostatic mechanisms, but circulating insulin is effective in lowering blood glucose only if there are sufficient insulin receptors to be activated. As body weight increases, the relative number of insulin receptors declines. The circulating insulin appears to be ineffective, and raised blood glucose levels result in a further rise in the circulating level of insulin (i.e. hyperinsulinaemia). This so-called 'syndrome X'[1] is characterized by obesity, hypertension, hyperlipidaemia and hyperinsulinaemia. Weight reduction reverses this situation by increasing the number of insulin receptors and improving glucose homoeostasis.

The breakdown of glucose homoeostasis may result from decreased insulin secretion caused by damage to the insulin-secreting pancreatic islet cells, or from insulin resistance due to an absolute decrease in the number of insulin receptors or (exceptionally) due to the presence of receptor antibodies. The severity of islet cell damage or insulin resistance determines the magnitude of the disturbance in glucose homoeostasis; a minor disturbance results in impaired glucose tolerance (IGT), but a more severe disturbance leads to the chronic hyperglycaemia diagnostic of diabetes.

In severe insulin deficiency, the patient develops not only hyperglycaemia (secondary to glycogen breakdown and glucose formation in the liver) but also ketoacidosis, which is the accumulation of acidic ketone bodies formed in the liver by incomplete oxidation of fatty acids, a process normally inhibited by insulin (see Chapter 10). In the absence of treatment, fatal diabetic ketoacidosis develops.

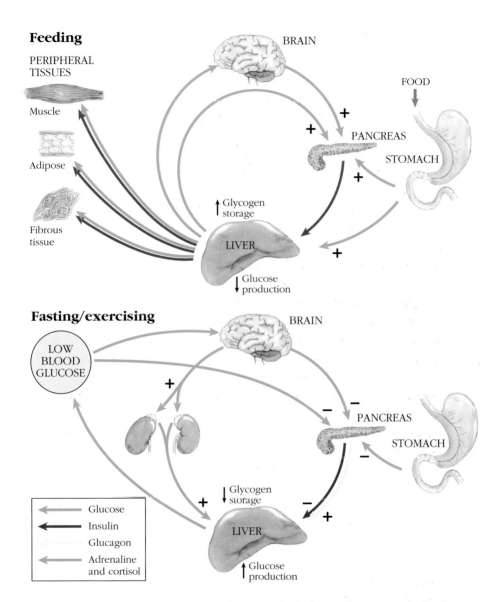

Figure 1.1 *Blood glucose homoeostasis in non-diabetic people. The hormonal responses to feeding, fasting and exercise interact to maintain the blood glucose level within a narrow range.*
Circulating insulin reduces glucose production (i.e. gluconeogenesis and glycogen breakdown) by the liver.
The reduction in circulating insulin, combined with increases in glucagon, cortisol and adrenaline (in response to fasting or exercise) increases glucose production (via gluconeogenesis and glycogen breakdown) in the liver.

Classification of the diabetes syndrome

The WHO classification of diabetes is now generally accepted (Table 1.1)[2]. The majority of patients fall into one of two classes, insulin dependent diabetes mellitus (IDDM) and non-insulin dependent diabetes mellitus (NIDDM), so most of this book is inevitably concerned with these two conditions. IDDM and NIDDM are the terms most commonly used nowadays, though they have also been referred to as Type I and

Table 1.1 WHO classification of diabetes mellitus and glucose intolerance[2]

Clinical classes

Diabetes mellitus
- Insulin dependent diabetes mellitus (IDDM)
- Non-insulin dependent diabetes mellitus (NIDDM)
  - Non-obese
  - Obese
- Malnutrition related diabetes mellitus (MRDM)
- Other types of diabetes mellitus associated with specific conditions and syndromes
- Gestational diabetes mellitus (see Chapter 12)

Impaired glucose tolerance (IGT)
- Non-obese
- Obese
- Associated with certain conditions and syndromes

Statistical risk classes
- Previous abnormality of glucose tolerance (e.g. past history of gestational diabetes or steroid induced diabetes)
- Potential abnormality of glucose tolerance (i.e. people at risk of diabetes, such as those with islet cell antibodies or with an identical twin who has IDDM)

Type II diabetes, respectively. In a few patients, diabetes is secondary to a clearly defined pathological process[3].

IDDM

IDDM is considered to be diabetes requiring insulin treatment within 3 months of diagnosis and/or with episodes of ketoacidosis (see Chapter 8 for management). The reliance on insulin treatment for survival distinguishes IDDM from NIDDM. Although IDDM usually arises before 40 years of age, IDDM with ketoacidosis can occur at any age.

NIDDM

This condition usually occurs after 40 years of age, though cases of maturity onset diabetes of the young (MODY) syndrome do arise. NIDDM may be subdivided into non-obese and obese types. Treatment with diet and, if necessary, oral hypoglycaemic agents, is generally satisfactory, though insulin treatment may be necessary to obtain good glycaemic control. The patient is not insulin dependent, however, as even with high blood glucose levels, there is no tendency to develop ketoacidosis.

NIDDM must never be interpreted as 'mild' diabetes, nor should patients be allowed to consider it so (see page 257). Although NIDDM may be successfully treated by dietary regulation alone (see Chapters 5 and 7), if ignored, it can maim and kill. The long-term complications of NIDDM are as severe and as prevalent as those of IDDM.

Causative factors for diabetes development

IDDM

The worldwide variation in the incidence of IDDM (from less than 1/100,000 in Japan to over 25/100,000 in Scandinavia) suggests a combination of genetic and environmental factors. IDDM is an autoimmune disease, which develops due to a breakdown in the normal immunological tolerance to the pancreatic β-cells.

Genetic factors: in 1994, a gene relating to pancreatic islet cell sensitivity to damage was discovered. It is unlikely, however, that a single individual gene will prove to be responsible for diabetes, as the disease is multifactorial in origin.

The risk of developing diabetes is increased if parents or siblings have the disease (Table 1.2). The genes HLA-DR3 and/or HLA-DR4 are far more common in patients with IDDM than in the general UK population (95% *vs* 40%) and each has an influence on, for example, the speed of development of the disease. Other non-major histocompatibility genes are also thought to be involved in IDDM[4].

Environmental factors are believed to act as triggers in people who are genetically susceptible to the development of IDDM. The most likely candidates appear to be certain viral infections (e.g. congenital rubella, the mumps virus, coxsackie B3 or B4). Such viruses either attack islet cells directly or, more likely, stimulate the immune system to produce antibodies that cross react with various components of the islet cell. Whatever the mechanism, patients may be under immune attack for a number of years before the clinical onset of IDDM[5] (see page 242).

NIDDM

NIDDM is clearly a heterogeneous group of disorders in which both genetic and environmental factors are at work.

Table 1.2 The lifetime risk of developing diabetes mellitus. Adapted from Vadheim CM, Rotter JI, 1992[4].

	IDDM	NIDDM	IGT
General population	1/500	1/40	1/20
Relatives of diabetic people			
■ Siblings	1/14	1/8	1/4
■ Monozygotic twin	1/3		

Genetic factors: the concordance rate for NIDDM in identical twins lies between 50% and 90%. The MODY syndrome has a strong genetic background, appearing in successive generations and affecting 40–50% of siblings, suggesting an autosomal dominant inheritance pattern.

Despite living in the same environment, different ethnic groups have a widely varying prevalence of NIDDM (Table 1.3), suggesting the involvement of genetic factors. Various genetic markers have been found associated with NIDDM (e.g. 'insulin' genes, such as the insulin receptor gene and the glucose transporter gene[6]). HLA antigens also appear to be associated with NIDDM in various ethnic groups (e.g. the Pima Indians).

Environmental factors: nutritional environmental factors are important in the development of NIDDM. Reduced growth in utero and in early life is strongly linked with IGT and NIDDM[7]. It is also linked with hypertension and hyperlipidaemia (Figure 1.2).

Table 1.3 Prevalence of NIDDM in different ethnic groups living in the same country*. Adapted from Bennett PH et al., 1992[6]

Country	Ethnic group	Age (years)	Prevalence (%)
Australia	Caucasian	≥ 25	3.4
	Aboriginal	≥ 20	15.6
Singapore	Chinese	≥ 18	4.0
	Malay		7.6
	Indian		8.9
USA	White	20–74	6.1
	Black		9.9
	Mexican		12.6
	Pima Indian	≥ 20	34.1

*Based on screening for diabetes using WHO criteria, 1985

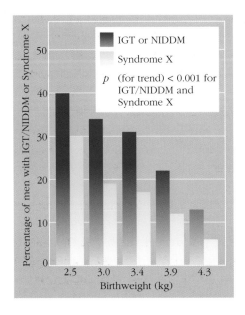

Figure 1.2 *Prevalence of IGT or NIDDM and syndrome X in men aged 64 years according to birthweight[7].*

Environmental factors play a significant role in determining the prevalence of diabetes. For example, Asian Indians who have migrated to many parts of the world show widely variable prevalences. In India the prevalence of NIDDM is 2.1% in the urban areas and 1.5% in rural populations; in Singapore, the prevalence is 8.9% and in South Africa 5%, compared to Fiji and Mauritius where the prevalence is 13%[6]. In the UK Southall survey of known diabetes, the prevalence of NIDDM in the resident Asian Indians aged 46–64 years was 2.2% – five times higher than in the Caucasian residents[8].

Diet and obesity: a definite correlation exists between the development of NIDDM, obesity, the proportion of fat in the diet, and the total energy intake. For example, Japanese sumo wrestlers, who consume 4500–6500 kcal/day, have a 40% chance of developing NIDDM and commonly die early from macrovascular disease. At times of a plentiful food supply, an increase in the incidence of obesity is associated with an increase in the incidence of the obese form of NIDDM. On the other hand, at times of diminished food supply, as observed during various wartime periods (e.g. in Holland during the 1939–45 war) both obesity and NIDDM show a decreased incidence. The incidence of NIDDM is directly proportional to the body mass index (BMI; body weight (kg)/height (m)^2), but those with a large waist:hip ratio for a given BMI have a higher risk of NIDDM development. Central obesity is for some reason particularly associated with IGT or diabetes, hypertension and hyperlipidaemia[6].

Other factors: the incidence of NIDDM increases with increasing age (Figure 1.3)[9].

An American study has shown a lower incidence of NIDDM among women who have regular modest exercise (at least 20 minutes three times a week) and that the protective effect of physical activity is independent of the other risk factors[10].

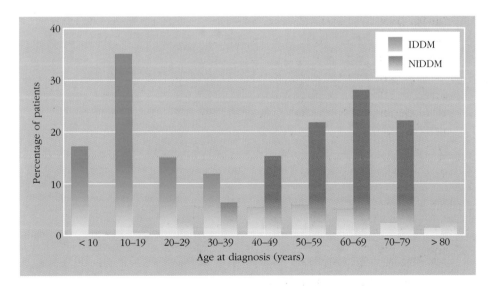

Figure 1.3 *Distribution of age at diagnosis according to type of diabetes. Reproduced with permission from Gatling W et al., 1988[9].*

Epidemiology

The prevalence of diagnosed diabetes is 1.5–2% in the UK and 2–3% in the adult population of the USA. However, screening usually identifies as many undiagnosed diabetic people in the community, suggesting a true prevalence of 4–6%[4]. The annual incidence of IDDM in children is 6–15/100,000, while the incidence of IDDM in the middle-aged and elderly is unknown.

The incidence of NIDDM is not well documented because of its insidious onset, but it has been estimated as 0.3/1000 people aged 20 years and over[4].

Secondary diabetes and MODY are uncommon, accounting for only 2% of cases of diabetes in the community.

Morbidity and mortality associated with diabetes

For diabetic patients, morbidity and mortality are considerably increased above those of the non-diabetic population.

■ The overall incidence of disability in diabetic patients is two or three times greater than that of non-diabetic people.

■ About 25% of all patients reaching end stage renal failure and requiring dialysis or transplantation have diabetes.

■ The most common single cause of end stage renal failure is now diabetes mellitus.

■ Diabetes mellitus is the most common single cause of blindness between the ages of 20 and 60 years in the UK.

■ Gangrene of the lower limbs, requiring amputation, is 20–30 times more common among diabetic patients than among non-diabetic people.

Diabetes mellitus causes a significant decrease in life expectancy (see page 69). The mortality from circulatory disease alone is twice that of matched non-diabetic people (see page 184). More recent cohort studies in IDDM have shown, however, that mortality has fallen significantly in the last 40 years[11]. Improved survival has been clearly shown to be associated with regular attendance at a diabetic clinic (Figure 1.4)[12]. The provision of regular diabetic care along with the move towards a shared care approach (see Chapter 3) represents an important method of reducing diabetes morbidity and mortality, which is the objective of the St Vincent Declaration[13].

The St Vincent Declaration

In October 1989, the European offices of the WHO and the International Diabetes Federation convened a meeting in St Vincent, Italy, which brought together patients with diabetes, their relatives, health care workers involved in diabetes management and politicians involved with the provision of resources. The outcome was a document known as the St Vincent Declaration[13]. This declaration states that it is within the power of national governments to create conditions in which a major reduction in the heavy burden of disease and death from diabetes can be achieved. At the core of this statement are a series of general recommendations and a number of specific clinical targets (Table 1.4). If the St Vincent targets are to be achieved, well organized and fully integrated diabetes care is essential.

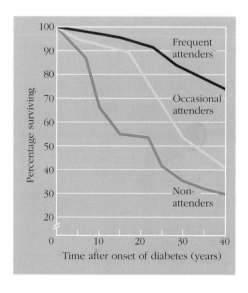

Figure 1.4 *Survival rates among diabetic patients according to their diabetic clinic attendance. Reproduced with permission from Deckert T et al., 1978*[12].

Table 1.4 The St Vincent Declaration[13]

General recommendations:

- Programmes for detection of diabetes and its complications
- Self care and community support for diabetes
- Raising of awareness that prevention of complications is possible
- Training and teaching in diabetes management
- Specialist facilities to manage diabetes in adults and children
- Necessary social, economic and emotional support for families of diabetic people
- Reinforcement and creation of centres of diabetes excellence
- Removal of hindrance to integration of people with diabetes in society

Specific clinical targets:

- Reduction of new blindness due to diabetes by one-third or more
- Reduction in numbers of people entering end stage renal failure by at least one-third
- Reduction by one-half of the incidence of leg amputations for diabetic gangrene
- Reduction in morbidity and mortality from coronary heart disease (not quantified)
- Achievement of pregnancy outcomes in women with diabetes equal to those of non-diabetic women

Is good control necessary?

The goals in treating diabetes may be summarized as follows:

- a happy and confident patient
- improved quality of life
- normal longevity.

The attainment of these goals necessitates a reduction in morbidity and mortality of diabetes, and this requires a considerable commitment not only from health care workers but also from patients. Health care workers tend to forget, in their efforts to reduce morbidity and mortality, the intrusion of diabetes in a patient's lifestyle. A holistic approach is essential. While juggling with medication to control glycaemia, blood pressure and lipid profiles, it should never be forgotten that the patient is a human being.

The Diabetes Control and Complications Trial (DCCT)[14] has finally confirmed that long-term complications can be reduced by good glycaemic control. The question is, how good does glycaemic control have to be and how is it best measured?

Measurement of glycaemic control: the assessment and management of diabetic patients was revolutionized by the discovery that glycated plasma proteins, such as fructosamine (a mixture of plasma proteins but mainly glycated albumin) and glycated haemoglobin (HbA_1 and HbA_{1C}) reflected mean plasma glucose concentrations over a period of time determined by the half-life of the protein in the body – 2 weeks for fructosamine and 2 months for glycated haemoglobin. Glucose in the blood combines reversibly with blood proteins and the products undergo irreversible rearrangement (Amadori reaction) to form permanently glycated proteins. The percentage of any protein that is glycated depends on the glucose concentration, the protein concentration, the period of time that glucose concentration is maintained and the lifetime of the protein in question. Red blood cells have a longer half-life than albumin, so glycated haemoglobin reflects the plasma glucose concentration over a longer period of time than fructosamine.

As there are several points on the haemoglobin molecule where glucose can become attached, there are several different glycated haemoglobins. All HbA_1 molecules have only one glucose/ haemoglobin but may be subdivided according to the point of attachment (e.g. HbA_{1C}). Some laboratories determine HbA_1, but these days more laboratories determine HbA_{1C}. As their methods vary, each laboratory has its own normal range (see page 137). Most diabetologists regard glycated haemoglobin as the preferred tool for assessing glycaemic control.

In certain conditions, interpretation of HbA_{1C} must be cautious, as it is affected by anaemia, increased red cell turnover and haemoglobinopathy. Similarly, fructosamine levels are falsely lowered by increases in plasma protein concentration and turnover, such as those occurring in pregnancy, nephrotic syndrome, chronic renal failure, chronic liver disease and inflammatory processes (e.g. rheumatoid arthritis). Successive HbA_{1C} determinations can give reliable information about the individual patient's level of glycaemic control.

The DCCT was a large trial involving 1441 patients and its aim was to see whether the tight glycaemic control achieved with intensive insulin therapy would prevent the development and progression of diabetic complications in patients with IDDM[14]. Patients were divided into two groups: one group treated conventionally (one or two insulin injections/day with little emphasis on blood glucose monitoring) and the other treated intensively (three or more insulin injections/day or continuous infusion from an insulin pump, plus frequent monitoring and insulin adjustment). The mean initial HbA_{1C} was 9%, as against a normal upper limit of 6.05%. Within 6 months, the HbA_{1C} in the intensively treated group dropped to 7.0% while in the conventionally treated group, the HbA_{1C} was 8.7%.

The effect of this improvement in glycaemic control on the primary prevention of long-term complications was clear cut and convincing after only 5 years of follow-up. The reduction in risk in the intensively treated group compared with the conventionally treated group was 76% for retinopathy development, 60% for neuropathy, and from 35–56% for nephropathy. Even when patients with early signs of a complication were considered, the risk of progression was reduced by intensive therapy. In secondary prevention of retinopathy the risk reduction was 47–54%, while for neuropathy, it was 60%, and for nephropathy, 50%.

Since the publication of the DCCT results, there has been considerable discussion concerning how good glycaemic control must be in order to minimize the risk of complications. Recent work on patients with IDDM has indicated that the relation between the prevalence of microalbuminuria and the degree of hyperglycaemia is non-linear (i.e. a threshold effect is seen at HbA_{1C} of 8.1%, above which the prevalence of microalbuminuria increases sharply)[15]. A threshold effect is also found for retinopathy but at a higher degree of hyperglycaemia. More work is needed in this area as the idea of thresholds is still unproven, but if they do exist, it has been suggested that a sensible target for physicians to aim for might be HbA_{1C} below 8.1% rather than as low as possible[16]. Tight control involves a greater risk of hypoglycaemia, and during the DCCT, it was found that in the intensively treated group, severe hypoglycaemia was three times more common than in the conventionally treated group.

It would be unwise to extrapolate the results of the DCCT to patients with NIDDM. The UK Prospective Diabetes Study (a 10-year follow-up of 4500 patients with NIDDM) should answer this question when it is completed in 1998. In the meantime, it is probably a sound assumption that good glycaemic control is good for patients with diabetes, whether with IDDM or NIDDM. It should always be borne in mind, however, that professionals involved in diabetes care are treating patients and not HbA_{1C} levels. As one patient once remarked, "Psychological and physical well-being are very important to us as patients but can sometimes be overlooked in favour of HbA_{1C}."

Shared care summary

■ Diabetes mellitus is a disease related to failure of glucose homoeostasis caused by a combination of genetic and environmental factors.

■ It is a heterogeneous group of conditions, most commonly classified as IDDM (or Type I) and NIDDM (or Type II).

■ The prevalence of diagnosed diabetes is 1.5–2.0% in the UK and 2–3% in the USA.

■ Patients with diabetes suffer considerable morbidity (from long-term complications) and premature mortality.

■ Glycated haemoglobin (HbA$_{1C}$) is a very useful measure of glycaemic control over a 2-month period.

■ Good glycaemic control has been shown to reduce the risk of developing complications in patients with IDDM (the American DCCT study).

■ Regular diabetes care, as opposed to intermittent or no care, is associated with a better outcome in terms of survival.

■ The St Vincent Declaration is a European initiative to improve international awareness of diabetes and promote better care.

References

1 Reaven GM. Role of insulin resistance in human disease. *Diabetes* 1988; **37:** 1595–607.

2 World Health Organisation. *Diabetes mellitus. Report of a WHO study group.* Technical Report Series 727. Geneva: WHO, 1985.

3 Harris MI, Zimmet P. Classification of diabetes mellitus and other categories of glucose intolerance. In: Alberti KGMM, DeFronzo RA, Keen H, Zimmet P, eds. *International textbook of diabetes mellitus.* Chichester, UK: John Wiley & Sons, 1992: 3–18.

4 Vadheim CM, Rotter JI. Genetics of diabetes mellitus. In: Alberti KGMM, DeFronzo RA, Keen H, Zimmet P, eds. *International textbook of diabetes mellitus.* Chichester, UK: John Wiley & Sons, 1992: 31–98.

5 Gorsuch AN, Spencer KM, Lister J, Wolf E, Bottazo GF, Cudworth AG. Can future Type 1 diabetes be predicted? A study in families of affected children. *Diabetes* 1982; **31:** 862–6.

6 Bennett PH, Bogardus C, Tuomilehto J, Zimmet P. Epidemiology and natural history of NIDDM: non-obese and obese. In: Alberti KGMM, DeFronzo RA, Keen H, Zimmet P, eds. *International textbook of diabetes mellitus.* Chichester, UK: John Wiley & Sons, 1992: 147–76.

7 Barker DJP. *Mothers, babies and disease in later life.* London: BMJ Publishing Group, 1994: 80–93.

8 Mather HM, Keen H. The Southall Diabetes Survey: prevalence of known diabetes in Asians and Europeans. *BMJ* 1985; **291:** 1081–4.

9 Gatling W, Mullee M, Hill RD. General characteristics of a community-based diabetic population. *Practical Diabetes* 1988; **5:** 104–7

10 Horton ES. Exercise and decreased risk of NIDDM. *N Engl J Med* 1991; **325:** 196–8.

11 McNally PG, Raymond NT, Burden ML *et al.* Trends in mortality of childhood-onset insulin-dependent diabetes mellitus in Leicestershire: 1940–1991. *Diabet Med* 1995; **12:** 961–6.

12 Deckert T, Poulsen JE, Larsen M. Prognosis of diabetics with diabetes onset before the age of thirty one. *Diabetologia* 1978; **14:** 371–7.

13 World Health Organisation (Europe) and International Diabetes Federation (Europe). Diabetes care and research in Europe: the Saint Vincent Declaration. *Diabet Med* 1990; **7:** 360.

14 The Diabetes Control and Complications Trial Research Group. The effect of intensive treatment of diabetes on the development and progression of long-term complications in insulin dependent diabetes mellitus. *N Engl J Med* 1993; **329:** 977–86.

15 Krolewski AS, Laffel LMB, Krolewski M, Quinn M, Warram JH. Glycosylated hemoglobin and the risk of microalbuminuria in patients with insulin-dependent diabetes mellitus. *N Engl J Med* 1995; **332:** 1251–5.

16 Viberti G. A glycemic threshold for diabetic complications? *N Engl J Med* 1995; **332:** 1293–4.

Further reading

Dowse G, Zimmet P. The thrifty genotype in non-insulin dependent diabetes. *BMJ* 1993; **306:** 532–3.

Nathan DM. Hemoglobin A_{1c} – infatuation or the real thing? *N Engl J Med* 1990; **323:** 1062–3.

Chapter 2

Diagnosing diabetes

Diabetes mellitus is an extremely common disease yet it often remains undiagnosed. This may be because the symptoms are mild or because the condition develops gradually over months or years. Opportunistic screening is easily carried out by the initial step of testing the urine for glucose. Subsequent steps in the diagnostic pathway are considered in this chapter. Finally, diagnosis of diabetes in a patient presenting with symptoms is discussed. The WHO diagnostic criteria based on the modified glucose tolerance test (GTT) are specified, and the standard method of carrying out the GTT, which is easily done in general practice, is described.

Screening for diabetes

Population screening

Screening for diabetes is seldom a routine procedure anywhere in the world. It is certainly not in the UK, even though the prevalence of undiagnosed non-insulin dependent diabetes (NIDDM) is thought to be similar to that of diagnosed NIDDM. A research study in Cambridgeshire, UK found that 4.5% of the 40–60-year-olds had undiagnosed NIDDM and 16.7% had impaired glucose tolerance (IGT)[1]. Although one might assume that early diagnosis and efficient management of NIDDM would decrease the morbidity and mortality of the disease, there is no published evidence to support this assumption. No significant benefit was found in a study carried out in

Bedford, UK in the 1960s[2], when after screening for NIDDM, patients were randomized to receive dietary advice plus either tolbutamide or placebo.

The benefits of good diabetic control in NIDDM remain unknown. Translation of the results of the Diabetes Control and Complications Trial (see page 14) to NIDDM is not acceptable because of the long periods of undiagnosed hyperglycaemia that commonly arise in NIDDM. Mortality in those with NIDDM is due mainly to macrovascular disease, which may be unaffected by good glycaemic control. People with IGT have an increased risk of macrovascular disease, yet their blood glucose levels are much lower than in many patients with treated NIDDM. The results of the UK Prospective Diabetes Study (see page 15) may answer the question concerning the benefit of good glycaemic control in NIDDM. If a significant benefit results from good control in NIDDM, active population screening programmes may prove to be justified. In addition, new trials are being organized to investigate whether early intervention in IGT and NIDDM will change the natural history of the disease.

Opportunistic screening

Diabetes is common and its prevalence is age related, so it makes sense to screen those who are at higher risk than the general population (Table 2.1). As urine testing for glucose is so simple, it may readily be incorporated into the general health screening checks carried out in general practice. The diagnostic pathway outlined in Figure 2.1 should be followed.

WHO diagnostic criteria for diabetes mellitus

Blood glucose levels in the general population show a continuous distribution. The division between normal and abnormal is arbitrary, but the WHO have published cut-off points based on sound scientific evidence (Table 2.2)[3].

Table 2.1 Factors associated with a higher than average risk of NIDDM

- Obesity (i.e. body mass index > 30 kg/m^2)
- Family history of NIDDM in first degree relative (i.e. parent, sibling or offspring)
- Hyperlipidaemia
- Hypertension
- Coronary artery disease
- Cerebrovascular disease
- Peripheral vascular disease
- Peripheral neuropathy
- History of gestational diabetes
- History of giving birth to a large baby (> 4 kg)
- History of skin infections (e.g. boils, whitlows, vaginal candidiasis, intertrigo)

Epidemiological research has defined a level of glucose intolerance that is associated with the development of diabetic complications. People with this level of intolerance or worse are defined as having diabetes, while those in the grey area between normal glucose tolerance and glucose intolerance typical of diabetes are said to have IGT. The significance and management of IGT are outlined in Table 2.3[4].

A method of carrying out a GTT, which has been standardized particularly with regard to glucose load, has been adopted worldwide, though different laboratories employ different samples (venous plasma or venous whole blood). WHO diagnostic criteria are available for each type of sample (Table 2.2).

Diagnosing diabetes in a patient with symptoms

Diabetes readily springs to mind when a patient presents with the classic symptoms of thirst, polyuria and weight loss. Several other

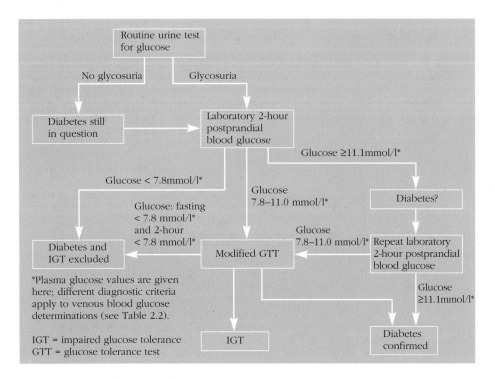

Figure 2.1 *Pathway for diabetes diagnosis in the absence of symptoms.*

symptoms (Table 2.4) may occur with diabetes or its complications. On suspicion of diabetes, the first step is to test a urine sample for glucose and ketones, followed by the sequence of steps outlined in Figure 2.2.

A finger-prick blood test is not sufficiently accurate for diagnostic purposes; in most cases, a single laboratory determination of plasma glucose in a 2-hour postprandial sample will suffice. In the past, fasting blood samples have been used to detect diabetes, but this method is not sufficiently sensitive; indeed, a screening study found that 50% of newly diagnosed diabetic patients had a normal fasting blood glucose[5].

Although urinary ketones may be due to prolonged fasting, they usually indicate IDDM and should be taken seriously. When

Table 2.2 WHO diagnostic criteria for diabetes and IGT[3*]

	Venous plasma	Venous whole blood
Diabetes mellitus		
Fasting glucose (mmol/l)	≥ 7.8 and/or	≥ 6.7 and/or
2-hour glucose (mmol/l)**	≥ 11.1	≥ 10.0
IGT		
Fasting glucose (mmol/l)	< 7.8 and	< 6.7 and
2-hour glucose (mmol/l)	7.8–11.0	6.7–10.0
Normal glucose tolerance		
Fasting glucose (mmol/l)	< 5.6 and	
2-hour glucose (mmol/l)	< 7.8	

*Criteria based on the modified GTT. Criteria vary according to the sample taken: venous plasma or venous whole blood.
**2 hours after 75g glucose taken by mouth

glycosuria and ketonuria are present in a child under 16 years of age, it is essential to contact a hospital paediatrician immediately, as ketoacidosis can develop within a few hours. In adults with IDDM, urgent referral is necessary — immediately for a dehydrated patient, and otherwise, within 24 hours by phone or fax. Such patients can usually be assessed within working hours and insulin treatment started at home with the help of a diabetes specialist nurse.

The majority of patients presenting with symptoms in general practice have NIDDM. As soon as the laboratory glucose result is available, the patient should be seen, informed and reassured. Simple dietary guidelines can be given straight away, though subsequent assessment and education may be organized either by referral to the hospital or within the general practice (see Chapter 3).

Patients who present with symptoms possibly due to diabetes but without accompanying glycosuria should have a laboratory 2-hour postprandial plasma glucose determination, and if this is not

Table 2.3 Diagnosis, management and prognosis of IGT[4]

Definition	Fasting plasma glucose < 7.8 mmol/l and 2-hour post-glucose load (75 g) plasma glucose 7.8–11.0 mmol/l
Significance	No development of microvascular diabetic complications but mortality and morbidity from cardiovascular disease is increased in comparison with general population
Natural history	After 10 years' follow-up: ■ 15% developed NIDDM ■ 22% remained with IGT ■ 53% improved to normal glucose tolerance
Management	■ Screen for and treat/advise on risk factors for cardiovascular disease (hypertension, hyperlipidaemia, obesity, smoking) ■ Review drug therapy; stop thiazides and β-blockers if possible ■ Advise low-sugar diet ■ Encourage regular physical activity ■ Organize annual plasma glucose estimation (ideally 2 hours postprandially) to detect progression to diabetes

diagnostic of diabetes, a modified GTT should be arranged. The GTT (Figure 2.3) can be carried out in general practice.

Getting the diagnosis right

Diabetes is an incurable, lifelong disease. It requires lifelong dietary compliance, regular monitoring, constant treatment and annual screening for complications. It leads to increased life insurance

Table 2.4 Symptoms suggestive of diabetes mellitus

- Urinary symptoms: polyuria, nocturia, urinary incontinence
- Thirst
- Weight loss
- Tiredness and irritability
- Rapid deterioration in visual acuity
- Boils, cellulitis or poor wound healing
- Fungal infections (e.g. vaginal candidiasis, balanitis, intertrigo)

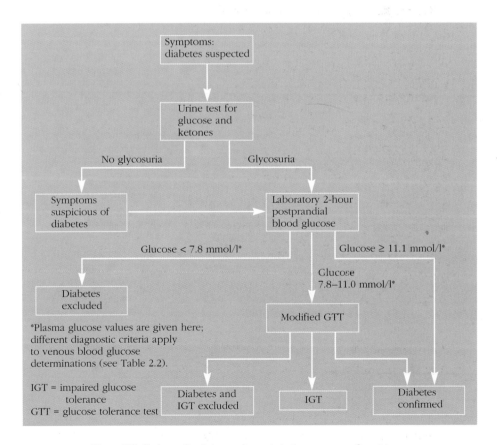

Figure 2.2 *Pathway for diabetes diagnosis in the presence of symptoms.*

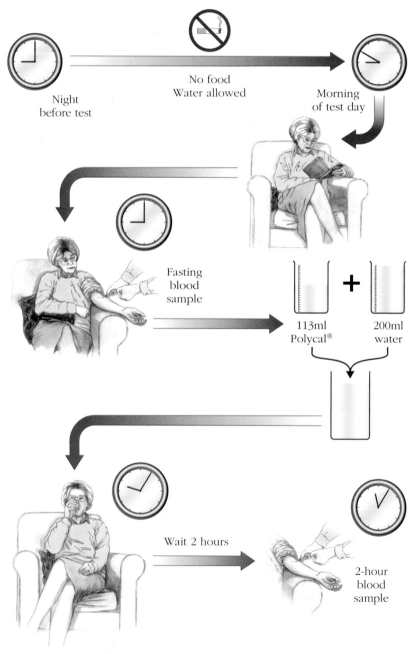

No food
Water allowed

Night
before test

Morning
of test day

Fasting
blood
sample

113ml
Polycal®

200ml
water

Wait 2 hours

2-hour
blood
sample

Figure 2.3 *Procedure for the modified GTT.*

Shared care summary

■ Diabetes mellitus is a lifelong disease with serious consequences. Accurate diagnosis in primary care is essential

■ Diagnosis of diabetes is made according to WHO diagnostic criteria. In primary care, a high index of suspicion and opportunistic screening is needed to diagnose diabetes.

■ Urine testing for glucose is the first step in diagnosis. If glycosuria is present, a laboratory plasma glucose (preferably 2 hours postprandial) should be taken to confirm the diagnosis.

■ The majority of patients diagnosed in primary care have NIDDM.

■ Patients presenting with symptoms and found to have glycosuria and urinary ketones are likely to have IDDM. They need immediate referral to hospital.

■ IGT does not have the same consequences as diabetes, but it is associated with an increased risk of cardiovascular disease.

premiums, restricted issue of a driving licence, and possible loss of employment (see chapter 6, pages 68–72). It is vital, therefore, that the diagnosis is made accurately. Neither urine testing nor finger-prick blood testing are sufficient; the diagnosis of diabetes must be confirmed by at least one laboratory blood glucose determination.

References

1 Williams DRR, Wareham NJ, Brown DC *et al*. Undiagnosed impaired glucose tolerance in the community: the Isle of Ely Diabetes project. *Diabet Med* 1995; **12:** 30–5.

2 Keen H, Jarrett RJ, McCartney P. The ten-year follow-up of the Bedford Survey (1962–1972): glucose tolerance and diabetes. *Diabetologia* 1982; **22:** 73–8.

3 World Health Organisation. *Diabetes mellitus. Report of a WHO study group.* Technical Report Series 727. Geneva: WHO, 1985.

4 Davies MJ, Gray IP. Impaired glucose tolerance. *BMJ* 1996; **312:** 264–5.

5 Forrest RD, Jackson CA, Yudkin JS. The abbreviated glucose tolerance test in screening for diabetes: the Islington Diabetes Survey. *Diabet Med* 1988; **5:** 557–61.

Chapter 3

The shared care concept

Diabetes, like several other chronic diseases, is common and has an increasing prevalence. It is no longer possible anywhere in the world, nor is it appropriate, for specialist doctors to take on the complete care of all diabetic patients. Many of the testing and monitoring procedures for diabetes care are within the scope of a multidisciplinary primary health care team (PHCT).

Diabetes is an ideal candidate for shared care between the primary and secondary health care sectors. In a UK survey carried out in 1991[1], diabetes care schemes accounted for 48% of all shared care schemes in operation. The practical design varied widely, and about one-third had been set up only since 1989.

What is shared care?

Shared care has been defined in many different ways, a recent definition[1] being, "the joint participation of hospital consultants and general practitioners in the planned delivery of care for patients with a chronic condition, informed by an enhanced information exchange over and above routine discharge and referral notices." This definition requires expansion when the chronic condition in question is diabetes; shared diabetes care involves input from a range of health care professionals (Figure 3.1), and a collaborative team approach is essential. The aims of a diabetes shared care programme are outlined in Table 3.1. Some would argue that the most important component of the team is the patient, who must undertake a responsible role in

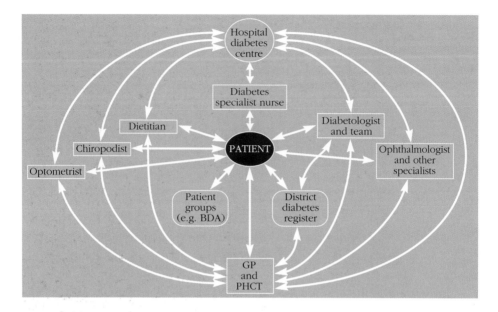

Figure 3.1 *Anatomy of a shared care scheme in the UK. The patient is central to the functioning of the professional shared care team, whose members may work in primary or secondary care or act as a bridge between the two.*

Table 3.1 Aims of a diabetes shared care programme

- Early and efficient diagnosis
- Identification and management of risk factors
- Weight monitoring and advice on diet
- Blood glucose control according to predefined targets
- Early detection and sound management of complications
- Prompt and appropriate referral for specialist advice
- Continual education and motivation of patients with diabetes
- Readily accessible care for all diabetic patients

BDA guidelines for patients

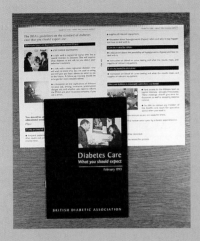

When you have just been diagnosed, you should have:

■ a full medical examination

■ a talk with a registered nurse who has a special interest in diabetes. She will explain what diabetes is and talk to you about your individual treatment

■ a talk with a state registered dietitian, who will want to know what you are used to eating and will give you basic advice on what to eat in the future. A follow-up meeting should be arranged for more detailed advice

■ a discussion on the implications of diabetes on your job, driving, insurance, prescription charges, etc. and whether you need to inform the DVLA and your insurance company, if you are a driver

■ information about the BDA's services and details of your local BDA group

■ ongoing education about your diabetes and the beneficial effects of exercise, and assessments of your control.

You should be able to take a close friend or relative with you to educational sessions if you wish.

Figure 3.2 *The patient's charter produced by the British Diabetic Association (BDA). Further guidelines on what to expect and on the role of the patient are included in the leaflet.*

the constant monitoring of his/her condition; to help patients understand the important aspects of diabetes care, the British Diabetic Association (BDA) issued guidelines on the care they should expect at diagnosis and follow-up (Figure 3.2). This chapter focuses on the roles of the professionals who provide this care.

Evolution of shared care systems

Shared care for diabetes is not a new concept, but was first tried as early as 1953 when a specially trained health visitor bridged the gap between an overworked hospital clinic and district nurses in general practice. By 1973, general practice based miniclinics were making an appearance[2]. Changes in the UK GP contract in 1990 and the institution of payment for chronic disease management in primary care in 1993, have led to 90% of primary care physicians in the UK claiming fees for diabetes care.

Over the past two decades, many types of shared care system for diabetes have been tried and tested in the UK. Greenhalgh[3] has systematically reviewed all of these systems, examining more than 50 schemes (over half of which were unpublished). Her main findings were as follows.

■ Established shared care schemes were of two types: centralized, hospital based and consultant led, or decentralized, community based and multidisciplinary.

■ A closely-knit steering group or an enthusiastic key individual, often the consultant diabetologist, could be clearly identified in all of the published successful schemes.

■ Structured care by primary care physicians with an interest in diabetes and supported by an enthusiastic specialist liaison team produced comparable and occasionally superior levels of care to those provided solely by the hospital diabetes department. Unstructured care was ineffective and wasteful of resources.

■ Three randomized, controlled trials showed that successful shared care schemes had two common features: a centralized prompting system, which recalled patients for appointments, and some form of structured checklist for the primary care physician.

■ Successful district-wide schemes shared three common features:
   an extensive planning phase when objectives were clearly defined and the facilities, expertise and commitment of primary care were assessed
   – locally developed, written guidelines for the management of diabetes
   – a well-developed outreach service from the hospital by highly trained nurse facilitators, who could advise on practical problems, maintain enthusiasm and enable fast tracking of patients for specialist review.

Several schemes have been reported in which patients receive routine care at a primary level and an annual review at the local hospital. Information is exchanged through cooperation cards kept by patients and letters, and overall administration and record keeping is achieved by central computer[4] (Figure 3.3). This model of integrated care has been found at least as effective as conventional hospital clinic care[5].

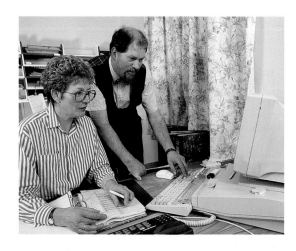

Figure 3.3 *Computerized record-keeping and administration.*

Another model of shared care involves initial education, assessment and management at the hospital diabetes department. Once stabilized, patients are transferred into primary care for long-term follow-up. If problems occur, specialist review is undertaken. Those with complications or unstable diabetes have their care undertaken either entirely by the hospital team or shared between the hospital and primary care. In this model, the burden of diabetes care in the district is shared between the primary and secondary sectors[6].

Is shared care effective?

Assessment of shared care schemes is certainly an undeveloped science as yet. Outcome parameters (e.g. good glycaemic control) and subjective but all important factors (e.g. patient satisfaction) are but two of the many aspects requiring assessment (see Chapter 18).

Results of diabetes follow-up in primary care in the early days of PHCTs' involvement were poor[7]. Some years later, one area published

---

Table 3.2 Advantages and disadvantages of shared care systems for diabetes

Advantages
- Continuity of care in familiar surroundings
- Holistic patient approach (including motivation, education and attention to cultural factors)
- Personal care from familiar health care personnel
- More accessible to patients
- More frequent monitoring
- Potential reduction in defaulters

Disadvantages
- No professional takes full responsibility
- Primary care less accustomed to routine follow-up
- PHCT may lack appropriate personnel
- PHCT members may lack expertise (e.g. in fundoscopy)

---

disappointing figures[8], though other groups are reporting better outcomes[4,5] and the debate on the effectiveness of shared care continues[9]. However, an enthusiastic PHCT and a cooperative spirit at the hospital diabetes department can make shared care work. Clearly, there is no universal recipe for shared care; the best models are developed through local cooperation.

Advantages of shared care

From the patient's point of view, involving the PHCT in diabetes care has advantages (Table 3.2). Care is continual, with the same familiar health care personnel, and it takes place predominantly in the local GP surgery. This approach encourages, for example, consideration of cultural issues (e.g. the avoidance of Friday afternoon clinics for muslims), and it gives the patient confidence to raise any points of concern. On the other hand, the expert specialist diabetes team is readily accessible should problems arise.

There are also advantages in shared diabetes care from the professional viewpoint; the expertise of the specialist team is employed effectively, yet all diabetic patients have access to high quality care in the primary sector. Areas of responsibility are clearly defined and any professional disadvantages are easily overcome by an enthusiastic PHCT willing to institute change and to seek continued professional training.

Shared care summary

Shared care for diabetes is still evolving in the UK, where contractual and financial changes in the NHS have contributed to its development. The essential components of a successful scheme for shared diabetes care are:

- careful tailoring to locality and resources
- extensive planning, with a negotiated contract involving agreed responsibilities and referral criteria

- an efficient, preferably computerized, prompting system for recalling patients

- a shared patient record system plus record cards/books for patients

- a written protocol for the PHCT

- educational support for the PHCT

- a well-developed outreach service from the hospital (e.g. involving nurse facilitators)

- an integral audit system involving primary and secondary care teams.

References

1 Hickman M, Drummond N, Grimshaw J. The operation of shared care for chronic disease. *Health Bull (Edinb)* 1994; **52:** 118–26.

2 Thorn PA, Russell RG. Diabetic clinics today and tomorrow: miniclinics in general practice. *BMJ* 1973; **ii:** 534–6.

3 Greenhalgh PM. *Shared care for diabetes: a systematic review.* Occasional paper 67. London: Royal College of General Practitioners, 1994.

4 Kopelman PG, Michell JC, Derrett CJ, Keast R, Sanderson A. A computerized system (DIASHARE) for the management and evaluation of diabetic care. *Diabet Med* 1992: **9:** S44.

5 Worth RC, Nicholson A, Bradley P. Shared care for diabetes in Chester: preliminary experience with a 'clinic-wide' scheme. *Practical Diabetes* 1990: **7:** 266–8.

6 Hill RD. Community care for diabetics in the Poole area. *BMJ* 1976; **i:** 1137–9.

7 Hayes TM, Harries J. Randomized controlled trial of routine hospital clinic care versus routine general practice care for Type 2 diabetes. *BMJ* 1984; **289:** 728–30.

8 Day JL, Humphreys H, Alban-Davies H. Problems of comprehensive shared diabetes care. *BMJ* 1987; **294:** 1590–2.

9 Sowden AJ, Sheldon TA, Alberti G. Shared care in diabetes. *BMJ* 1995; **310:** 142–3.

Chapter 4

Teaching people about diabetes

It is universally recognized that the need for education of patients about diabetes and its management is paramount. One of the most significant advances in diabetes care has been the recognition that the most important person in the diabetes care team is the patient, who needs to be empowered to take responsibility for his/her own health care rather than relying on others. Such empowerment involves the provision of education matched to the patient's abilities and capacity to learn.

This chapter sets out the aims of diabetes education and discusses the organizational strategy, including planning and teaching methods. The use of various types of audiovisual media is reviewed and the content of suitable education programmes outlined. In the UK, the major part of the educational process may be carried out in the primary or the secondary sector, depending on local policy and facilities.

Breaking the news of the diagnosis

Only when the diagnosis of diabetes has been confirmed should the patient be told. The news of the diagnosis should preferably be conveyed by someone who is known to the patient (e.g. the family practitioner or the practice nurse). The emotional response to this news can range from relief to total devastation, and it may be clouded by memories of other people with diabetes who are known to the patient. A knowledgeable and positive approach by the health care professionals is necessary for successful long-term management of diabetes.

When is education appropriate?

The person with newly diagnosed diabetes has to pass through the grief reaction (Figure 4.1) before accepting the disease. The time course of achieving a healthy state of acceptance varies with each individual. For some people, the grieving process may never be completed, and those patients will remain at the stage of anger or denial.

The timing of education is very important and will vary from patient to patient, depending on age at diagnosis, type of diabetes, level of intelligence and the relevant stage in the grief reaction. It is not wise, and it may even be counterproductive, to overburden the patient and family with information too soon after diagnosis.

Aims of education

The aims of education are to encourage patients to accept responsibility for their own health care, to acquire the necessary information, both from education and from personal experience, and to alter their behaviour in the light of the acquired information. Education is the key to improved quality of life for the person with diabetes, and patients themselves are now expecting to be educated. Some health care professionals believe that education is a luxury that can be ill-afforded. Patient education may, however, improve self-care, help in the avoidance of complications and reduce hospital admissions.

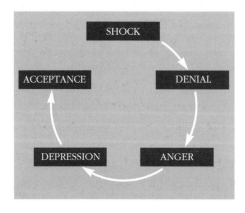

Figure 4.1 *The grief reaction.*

Organizational strategy

The educators

All members of the hospital-based diabetes team and the primary health care team (PHCT) should be involved as educators; a coordinated approach is helpful. It is important that all the educators speak with one voice and convey consistent messages. While an organized programme is useful, some patients require an individualized approach. All patients may be educated opportunistically, when they are particularly receptive.

Educational strategies

Health care professionals involved in the education of diabetic patients must be aware of the basic principles outlined in Table 4.1.

Teaching methods

Different teaching methods suit different types of patient at different stages in the history of their condition. Some patients learn quite happily in groups, while in certain situations, individual tuition is necessary. Group sessions have certain advantages; they foster interaction between patients and team members. Meeting others in a similar situation and sharing experiences can be reassuring (Figure 4.2).

Educational media

Verbal information: time taken to talk about diabetes is time well spent, and a discussion or two-way conversation is far better than a lecture. Verbal information is easily forgotten, however, and it needs reinforcement from other media.

Written information should be provided with visual images to help recall. Posters, leaflets and booklets are available from patient organizations, such as the British Diabetic Association. Patients need sound motivation to read these leaflets, and they also need to be able to read; illiteracy may be cleverly hidden from the educator, or English may not be the first language.

Table 4.1 The basis of successful diabetes education

- Patients are people who happen to have diabetes. They vary in age, learning ability, psychological profile, motivational qualities and degree of support from family and friends.
- Family members and/or carers should be included in the education programme so that they can become helpful cooperators rather than helpless bystanders.
- The idea of a partnership between patient and professional can help to maintain the patient's self esteem.
- The education programme should not merely inform, but should encourage patients to learn from experience and use the information they receive in their daily lives. Fear-arousing messages should be avoided.
- A balance is needed between theoretical instruction and practical advice. Patients need to be convinced that it is in their own best interests to modify their behaviour.
- Overloading should be avoided. Essential points may be obscured if surplus information is provided.
- Simple straightforward language is essential. Jargon and complex terminology can cause confusion.
- Patient education is a perpetual process. Review, repetition and reinforcement are vital components of successful education.

Audiovisual aids: a wide range of educational programmes on slides, audio-tapes or video is available. When selecting audiovisual aids, the needs of particular patients should be borne in mind. The content should be appropriate, and the presentation succinct and at the correct level. Before use, aids should be checked to ensure they are simple, appropriate and up-to-date, that the messages are consistent with those being given by other members of the diabetes care team and that they are technically satisfactory (i.e. legible, playable).

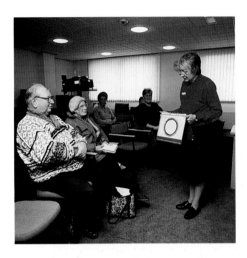

Figure 4.2 *A patient education session in a diabetes education centre.*

Educational programme content

Shortly after diagnosis, the patient comes into contact with doctors, nurses, dietitians, chiropodists and many others, including other patients with diabetes. It is essential that all the professional contacts convey similar information, views and attitudes; they should be consistent in every way. Understanding, empathy and enthusiasm should be universal but, above all, health care workers should convey optimism and a firm belief that an improved standard of health and well being is attainable.

Topics for consideration in a typical education programme are outlined in Table 4.2. The programme should be tailored to suit the needs of individual patients or groups.

Patient motivation

Some people are self-motivated both to learn about their diabetes and to take action to control it, even if this means considerable behavioural adaptation. Others need motivating by people or events, and it is here that the diabetes team has an important role to play. This motivation then needs reinforcing at intervals, when patients know what they should do, but fail to do it. Lack of motivation nullifies the best educational programme and the work of the most dedicated teachers.

Table 4.2 Topics for a diabetes educational programme

Topic*	Content
For all patients:	
1 Reassurance	Dispelling common misconceptions and fears
2 What is diabetes?	Insulin and the functions of the pancreas; hyperglycaemia and symptoms
3 Predisposing factors	Genetics, family history, surplus body weight, intercurrent illness, pregnancy, medication, pancreatic surgery or disease
4 General introduction to diabetes treatment	Education/information, exercise, healthy eating, tablets, insulin
5 Monitoring	Urine testing/blood glucose monitoring. Even the simplest monitoring procedures demand acceptance, motivation and commitment from the patient
6 Diet in detail	Individual dietary assessment and planning with a dietitian
7 Chiropody	Advice on daily foot care and hygiene; individual assessment by a chiropodist and referral for treatment
8 Diabetic control	**Why it is important:** to delay or alleviate complications, to avoid unpleasant symptoms (e.g. thirst and tiredness) **What affects it?** Adherence to recommended treatment, stresses of everyday life

	How is it measured? Weight, urine glucose, blood glucose levels, glycated haemoglobin
9 Follow-up	Advice on the need for regular checks, how often they are needed and where they can be carried out
10 Living with diabetes	Illness, other medication, education, medicolegal (employment, driving, insurance), holidays, sports and exercise, smoking, alcohol, eating out, marriage, contraception, pregnancy, impotence, menstruation
For insulin-treated patients:	
11 Insulin treatment	Types of insulin, syringes and pens, injections, storage, sharps disposal, dose adjustment
For patients treated with insulin or oral hypoglycaemic agents:	
12 Hypoglycaemia	Recognizing symptoms, avoiding hypos, treatment, loss of symptoms

*These are not the titles to be used for patients.

What is the best way to motivate patients? Fear-arousing messages about future complications are unlikely to be productive. It is helpful to concentrate on a few realistic, short-term objectives. For example, rather than telling the patient to lose 10 kg, it may be more productive to agree on a target weight for two months ahead (as a first step). Objectives should be precise, practical and achievable; they should be measurable and agreed with the patient.

The team must be ready to accept failure to reach the set targets without any negative judgemental comments. The golden rule is always to find something – anything – to praise, encourage or welcome. Finally, the team must realize that it is the patients' prerogative how much time and effort they spend on improving their own health. Their decisions may alter with time. Meanwhile, rejection of advice has to be respected and tolerated, even if it cannot be condoned.

Shared care summary

■ General education about diabetes is a perpetual process in which the PHCT plays a major role.

■ News of the diagnosis should be given by someone known to the patient.

■ At diagnosis, patients usually progress through a grief reaction before accepting their condition.

■ Education is as important for those with NIDDM as for those with IDDM. Patients with IDDM, although being referred to hospital for education about insulin treatment, also need the support of the PHCT.

■ It is important not to overburden patients with too much information at one time.

■ Motivating patients to take responsibility for their own care is integral to the education process.

Further reading

*†British Diabetic Association. *Balance for beginners. Starting out with diabetes (insulin dependent diabetes)*. London: British Diabetic Association, published annually.

*†British Diabetic Association. *Balance for beginners. Starting out with diabetes (non insulin dependent diabetes)*. London: British Diabetic Association, published annually.

Diabetes Education Study Group of the European Association for the Study of Diabetes. Survival kit: the 5-minute education kit. A document for health care providers and patients. *Diabet Med* 1995; **12:** 1022–43.

†Hillson R. *Diabetes: a young person's guide*. London: Optima, Little, Brown & Co., 1993.

National Association of Health Authorities and Trusts. *Health care for black and minority ethnic people*. NAHAT Briefing Issue 100. Birmingham: NAHAT, 1996.

†Sönksen P, Fox C, Judd S. *Diabetes at your fingertips. The comprehensive diabetes reference book for the 1990s. 2nd edn*. London: Class Publishing, 1991.

Stillitoe R. *Counselling people with diabetes*. Leicester: British Psychological Society BPS Books, 1994.

*The British Diabetic Association supply many other useful publications for both patients and professionals. Write to The British Diabetic Association, 10 Queen Anne Street, London W1M 0BD for a catalogue.

†Written for patients but may prove a useful resource for professionals.

Chapter 5

Healthy eating for diabetes

The views of health professionals on the nature of a healthy diet for diabetes have changed remarkably over the past two decades. The traditional view was that a disorder of carbohydrate metabolism merited a low-carbohydrate diet. When such a view was questioned in the 1970s, research was initiated on the effects of a high-carbohydrate/low-fat diet as opposed to a low-carbohydrate/high-fat and high-protein diet. The results prompted a dramatic change in dietary recommendations for diabetic patients (recently updated in the UK[1]).

The present recommendations for a good diet for people with diabetes mirror those of healthy eating promoted for the rest of the population and are, therefore, easier for diabetic patients to follow, provided that they are well informed.

Assessing the patient's basic knowledge and providing appropriate information should be undertaken by the dietitian soon after diagnosis of diabetes and may require several interviews. The dietitian's workload does not permit constant review of all patients with diabetes. Follow-up must be shared between the health care teams in both hospital and general practice. Thus, many dietary questions may be dealt with by other members of the team, who require a sound basic knowledge. Detailed dietary reviews by a dietitian are helpful every 3–5 years or when problems arise.

This chapter surveys the elements of diabetes dietary care in terms of education, motivation and monitoring, and considers how this care might be shared in order to satisfy the best interests of the patient.

Dietary recommendations

Aims of dietary treatment

The main aims of a healthy diet in the treatment of diabetes are:

- to abolish the primary symptoms by promoting normoglycaemia while ensuring optimal nutrition
- to minimize the risk of hypoglycaemia in those patients treated with insulin or oral hypoglycaemic agents (OHAs)
- to achieve and maintain ideal body weight/body mass index (BMI; see page 77)
- to minimize the risk of long-term microvascular and macrovascular complications.

In the UK, the current recommendations[1] are:

- eat regular meals
- eat more high-fibre carbohydrate foods
- eat less sugar and sugary foods
- cut down the amount of fat consumed
- avoid being overweight
- avoid special diabetic products
- reduce salt intake
- keep alcohol intake moderately low.

Energy consumption should not exceed requirements and, for weight loss, should be reduced below requirements. Weight loss in overweight patients with non-insulin-dependent diabetes (NIDDM) has been associated with increased life expectancy, while energy restriction in such patients abolishes primary symptoms even before weight loss is evident.

These recommendations are fairly straightforward from the point of view of health care professionals. They may need clarifying for patients, who need teaching clearly what they should do and motivating to do it. Motivation is a continuing process (see page 41), which members of the primary health care team (PHCT) are in a good position to accomplish and monitor. A miniclinic run by a trained practice nurse can successfully keep a check on weight, diet and patient morale. When recommending dietary change, personal and cultural preferences require careful consideration. Dietary advice may need adjusting in the light of religious rules on eating and fasting. Educational material specially prepared for ethnic minorities is available through patient organizations, such as the British Diabetic Association (BDA).

Weight reduction

Patients with NIDDM are often obese at presentation. A restriction of calorie intake and the accompanying weight loss often results in disappearance of symptoms of hyperglycaemia and improved glycaemic control.

Appropriate BMI targets are presented on page 77. Weight loss targets should be realistic and attainable and sustained weight loss of the order of 1–2 lb/week (0.5–1.0 kg/week) represents good progress. Diets that are too low in energy may cause the patient to make up the deficit with inappropriate foods. Commercially available very-low-calorie diets are inadvisable, as they may increase the risk of cardiac arrhythmias in patients with unrecognized heart disease.

An estimate of basal metabolic rate (BMR) and daily energy expenditure, based on sex, weight and activity level (Table 5.1), will confirm that the chosen calorie intake is below that for weight maintenance. It should be remembered, however, that overweight diabetic patients with NIDDM have higher energy requirements than expected from their ideal body weight.

Patients with IDDM who find weight control difficult should be discouraged from drastic dieting because of the dangers of hypoglycaemia. A suitable diet should consist of fewer calories than are required for weight maintenance and the carbohydrate should be spread evenly throughout the day. Insulin doses need to be reduced.

Table 5.1 Estimation of daily energy expenditure and weight loss based on BMR and activity level[2]

Consider a 50-year-old man who is an office worker.
Body weight 82 kg.
BMR = (11.6 x 82) + 879 = 1830 kcal/day*
Energy expenditure = BMR x Activity factor = 1830 x 1.55 (for light activity) = 2837 kcal/day

*Factors used in this equation can be found in reference 2.

Therefore, a daily intake of only 2200 kcal/day represents underprovision of 4460 kcal/week, which is equivalent to nearly 500 g of fat. Total weight reduction should be slightly over 1 lb/week.

The diet programme should be negotiated between doctor, patient and dietitian.

Components of the recommended diet

The proportions of carbohydrate, fat and protein in the diet recommended for diabetic patients (and indeed for the population as a whole) are outlined in Figure 5.1. For patients, these percentages should be converted into foods (Figure 5.2).

Carbohydrate: starchy high-fibre foods should form the basis of every meal and similar amounts should be eaten every day. Postprandial glucose absorption is then relatively slow and dramatic fluctuations are prevented.

Sugar need not be avoided completely, but should be eaten in only small quantities and along with high-fibre meals. Good artificial sweeteners are widely available, along with a growing variety of low-sugar jams and desserts.

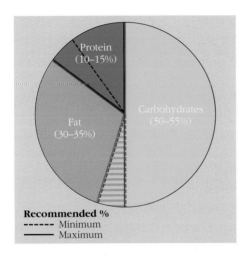

Figure 5.1 *Components (as percentage of total energy) of the currently recommended diet for diabetic patients in the UK[1].*

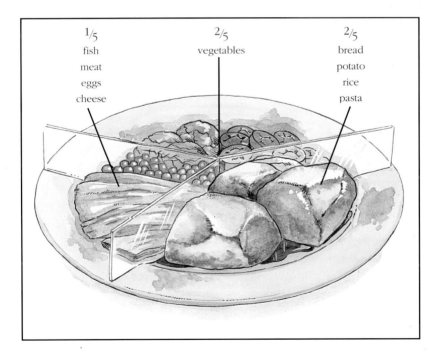

Figure 5.2 *Foods recommended for diabetic patients: the emphasis is on unrefined, high-fibre carbohydrates and fresh fruit and vegetables. Protein from meat, fish and dairy foods should be limited and should be accompanied by as little fat as possible.*

Fat: the major factor influencing serum cholesterol, and total and LDL cholesterol in particular, is saturated fat consumption rather than cholesterol intake *per se*. A reduction in saturated fat intake is important, particularly for patients with NIDDM. Limiting the consumption of fatty foods (such as butter, pastry, fatty meat and full-fat dairy products), and substituting the low-fat varieties, should reduce serum cholesterol and return the lipid profile towards normal. Patients are often unaware how much saturated fat is present in seemingly harmless snacks, such as crisps or plain biscuits (Table 5.2). Dietitians should suggest alternatives.

Polyunsaturated fat (common in sunflower oil, corn oil and soya oil) is often substituted for saturated fat when intake of the latter is to be reduced. This should be done only in moderation as a high intake of these oils, which is associated with lipid peroxidation, has been linked with heart disease[3], particularly if the diet is low in antioxidant-containing fruits and vegetables. Four to five servings of fruits and vegetables/day are recommended for people with diabetes, particularly if their intake of polyunsaturated fat is high.

The incidence of heart disease is low in Mediterranean countries, where monounsaturated fat (e.g. in olive oil) is consumed routinely. Although this may be coincidental, the use of monounsaturated fat (also found in rapeseed and peanut oil) is now being encouraged as an alternative to saturated and polyunsaturated fat.

Fish oils, which are rich in a certain type of fatty acids (long chain ω-3 fatty acids), appear to have beneficial effects on serum triglycerides. An increase in consumption of oily fish is, therefore, encouraged, though fish oil supplements are not recommended for people with diabetes as their use is still experimental and large doses have been shown to aggravate hyperglycaemia and elevate serum LDL cholesterol[4].

Protein: protein consumption should be modest. Reducing protein rich foods naturally reduces saturated fat intake, while substitution of plant protein sources (cereals and pulses) enables guidelines on dietary fibre to be met. Reducing protein intake has been shown to retard the progression of diabetic nephropathy[5].

Table 5.2 Comparative fat and carbohydrate contents of common snacks

Snack	Energy (kcal)	Fat (g)	Carbohydrate (g)
Wholemeal scone	158	5	26
Currant bun/teacake	148	4	26
1 slice bread + low-fat spread	80	3	10
1 slice malt loaf	94	1	20
Bowl of cereal + semi-skimmed milk	140	2	25
Cereal bar	150	7	20
Digestive biscuit	70	3.0	10
Ginger nut biscuit	46	1.5	10
Garibaldi biscuit	40	1	8
Banana	95	0.3	20
Diet yogurt	50	0.3	10
Vegetable samosa	163	7	21
Bhajia/Pakoras (140 g)	252	12	29
Bombay mix (25 g)	126	8	9
Pancake roll (60 g)	130	8	13
Crisps (30 g)	163	11	16

Salt: daily salt intake should be limited to 6 g or, for those with hypertension, 3 g. Reducing salt intake from 12 g/day to 6 g/day has been shown to reduce blood pressure[6], and this would be expected to be associated with a decreased risk of heart disease and stroke.

Diabetic foods: a subcommittee of the BDA has concluded that there is no need for diabetic foods in modern diabetes management and that their consumption may even be counterproductive when striving for good diabetic control[7]. These foods tend to be high in fat and to contain fructose as sweetener. Fructose should be avoided by poorly controlled patients. High fructose consumption may lead to undesirable fasting triglyceride levels, though this issue remains unresolved.

Alcohol: the medically recommended restriction on alcohol intake for diabetic patients is the same as for the rest of the UK population, viz. 2 units/day for women and 3 units/day for men[8]. One of the major problems caused by alcohol consumption in diabetic patients treated with insulin or OHAs is hypoglycaemia, which may be triggered by the inhibition of gluconeogenesis by alcohol. Certain beers, promoted as being suitable for diabetic people, are particularly inadvisable, because although they contain less carbohydrate than ordinary beers, they also contain more alcohol (e.g. 7.5%). Patients should drink alcohol only with or after a meal. If consumed regularly, the calorie content needs to be considered, particularly by those patients aiming to reduce body weight.

Monitoring carbohydrate consumption

Weighing and measuring carbohydrate foods, although encouraged in the past, is not necessary for good diabetic control. Factors other than the amount of carbohydrate may govern the rise in blood glucose in response to a meal (e.g. the amounts of dietary fibre, fat and protein in the meal and the physical form of the food). Meal planning is probably a more sensible approach to the management of carbohydrate consumption. Not only the content but also the timing of the meal is important for patients treated with insulin or OHAs, if hypoglycaemia is to be avoided. Appropriate foods for treatment of hypoglycaemia are described in Chapter 9.

Although exercise is encouraged in diabetic patients, its effects on the blood glucose level need to be considered. If glycaemic control is poor and the insulin supply is insufficient, glucose uptake is slow. Adrenaline released in response to physical activity stimulates glucose release from the liver and thus elevates blood glucose. If glycaemic control is good, physical activity increases the uptake of glucose by muscle and this may result in hypoglycaemia. Extra carbohydrate (e.g. 2 slices of bread or 4 oz potato) should be eaten at the meal prior to exercise and rapidly absorbed 'top-ups' (glucose drinks or tablets) may be required before and/or during exercise, if strenuous. As the hypoglycaemic effect of exercise can last for several hours, more unrefined carbohydrate should be eaten after the activity.

Education and motivation

Patients need constant advice on diet and the motivation to follow it. A simple explanation of the information commonly presented on food labels might also be helpful. The education process will probably be initiated by the dietitian and continued by the PHCT. Dietary advice must be tailored to the individual and cause minimal disruption to daily life. It must be understood by the patient, who should not be overburdened by too much information on one occasion. Repetition of important information, preferably with support from visual aids, such as leaflets and videos, is necessary if newly acquired knowledge is to be retained.

Motivation, which waxes strong initially, soon tends to wane and needs continual maintenance. For weight loss, regular group meetings provide support among patients who share a common goal. Recipes are another way of maintaining interest in diet and educating patients. Dietitians may produce recipe leaflets for patients at hospital outpatient clinics, and they might also consider distributing them to practice nurses in the area. Recipes for ethnic minority populations also need consideration in some areas.

Patients often receive apparently conflicting advice from the media and may wish to discuss points of confusion. Regular attendance at a practice miniclinic or slimming group organized by the practice nurse provides opportunities for discussing dietary problems and also for monitoring patients' weight.

Education for the PHCT is as important as education for the patients, and it may be accomplished by regular study days and training sessions held by the dietitian at the local hospital or diabetes centre, or by the community dietitian. Ideas may be pooled on methods of maintaining patients' interest and motivation.

The primary aim for dietitian, practice nurse and clinicians must be to encourage patients to eat and enjoy their food for general good health rather than considering it as a diet for treatment of disease, and to do this in such a way that body weight and blood glucose levels remain as stable and as near normal as possible.

Shared care summary

■ All newly diagnosed patients with diabetes should be referred to a state registered dietitian, who can assess their knowledge and provide appropriate information.

■ Dietary care is subsequently shared between the hospital and the PHCT.

■ All patients with diabetes mellitus benefit from review by a dietitian every 2–5 years.

■ Dietitians working with the PHCT should be well integrated into the scheme for provision of diabetes care.

■ The practice nurse may supervise weight loss in patients with NIDDM, possibly at miniclinics. She can also keep a check on diet, provide information and motivate the patient. Group meetings may be helpful.

■ The dietitian at the hospital may see patients, particularly those with IDDM, when they attend the outpatient clinic and may reinforce dietary information and maintain patient interest.

References

1 Nutrition Sub-committee, British Diabetic Association. Dietary recommendations for people with diabetes: an update for the 1990s. *Diabet Med* 1992; **9:** 189–202.

2 FAD/WHO/UNO. *Energy and protein requirements.* WHO Technical Report Series 724. Geneva: WHO, 1985: 397.

3 Gramenzi A, Gentile A, Fasoli M, Parrazzini F, Vecchia CL. Association between certain foods and risk of myocardial infarction in women. *BMJ* 1990; **300:** 771–3.

4 Axelrod L. Omega-3 fatty acids in diabetes mellitus: a gift from the sea? *Diabetes* 1989; **38:** 539–43.

5 Zeller K, Whittaker E, Sullivan L, Raskin P, Jacobson HR. Effect of restricting dietary protein on the progression of renal failure in patients with insulin dependent diabetes. *N Engl J Med* 1991; **324:** 78–84.

6 Intersalt Cooperative Research Group. An international study of electrolyte excretion and blood pressure. *BMJ* 1988; **297:** 319–28.

7 Nutrition Sub-committee, British Diabetic Association. Discussion paper on the role of diabetic foods. *Diabet Med* 1992; **9:** 300–6.

8 Connor H, Marks V. Alcohol and diabetes. *Diabet Med* 1985; **2:** 413–6.

Chapter 6

Living with diabetes

Management of diabetes by the patient involves coping with normal everyday activities. Patients need advice on keeping a check on their diabetic control, on what to do about legal matters, such as driving and employment, about life insurance, travel and holidays, and what to do if they develop a cold or a stomach upset. Sick day rules are covered in Chapter 10 (page 122); this chapter considers all these other aspects of diabetes management from both the patient and health care professional viewpoints.

Home monitoring of diabetes

All patients benefit from home monitoring of their diabetes – learning how their diabetes is affected by different activities and situations. Home monitoring records should be reviewed at each clinic visit and help given in their interpretation.

At first, monitoring is a novelty, but as the years go by, some patients forget to carry out tests regularly or they stop altogether. This is human nature, and health care professionals should try to encourage rather than scold. Monitoring generally stops because of poor motivation or lack of understanding of the significance of the results.

Why home monitoring?

Good diabetic control is now accepted as a valid means of reducing the risk of long-term complications; home monitoring is an essential part of achieving it. Symptoms are not useful indicators of poor control. Thirst and polyuria occur only when blood glucose levels are running consistently at more than twice normal values (10–20 mmol/l or higher). Many patients with poor control have no symptoms. They have often gradually slipped into this condition, and it is only when they later achieve good control that they recognize their past poor state of health.

The advantages of home monitoring are that:

■ it aids day-to-day self management
■ it gives early warning of poor control
■ it helps some patients to avoid hypoglycaemia
■ it helps to explain laboratory results.

Which method of monitoring?

Two basic methods of home monitoring are available: urine testing and finger-prick blood glucose testing. Both methods can be useful; the choice depends on the objectives set for the patient and the patient's capabilities.

Urine testing

This technique is quick and easy but has the disadvantage (Table 6.1) of reflecting only the overall level of control achieved since the bladder was last emptied. Urine tests are negative as long as the blood glucose level remains below the renal threshold (Figure 6.1). This would represent good diabetic control for the patient treated by diet with or without oral hypoglycaemic agents (OHAs). Urine testing is the preferred method for this group of patients. Some insulin treated patients may also choose this method because of its simplicity.

A few patients have a low renal threshold for glucose. In such patients, urine testing may show glycosuria despite good laboratory results. Some elderly patients have a high renal threshold. All home monitoring results may then be negative but laboratory results indicate poor control. Patients with an abnormal renal threshold may benefit from switching to blood glucose monitoring.

Table 6.1 Urine testing for glucose by diabetic patients

Advantages	Disadvantages
■ Inexpensive	■ Retrospective
■ Non-invasive and painless	■ Affected by renal threshold
■ Simple to carry out	■ Cannot detect hypoglycaemia
■ Gives early warning of deteriorating control in most patients	■ Poor indicator of actual blood glucose level
	■ Result affected by time since voiding

How to test: A variety of urine testing strips are available in the UK (Table 6.2). The testing technique, which can be found in manufacturer's instructions with the test strips, should be carefully taught. Accurate timing is essential.

Tests should be undertaken once a day but varying the time of day (i.e. on rising in the morning, before lunch, before the evening meal, 2 hours after a main meal and before bedtime). Over several days, this type of monitoring gives some idea of control throughout the day and demonstrates when treatment needs to be modified to improve control. Ideally, all urine tests should be negative.

Home blood glucose monitoring (HBGM)

The advent of HBGM has revolutionized the care of insulin-treated diabetic patients and strongly contributes to patients' independence and self management. Many patients quickly master the technique and find the results educational. It helps patients to gain control over their diabetes and to continue with a wide range of daily activities.

HBGM also has significant disadvantages (Table 6.3), which may discourage many patients. Recommending HBGM is not only concerned with teaching the patient how to do the test, but also

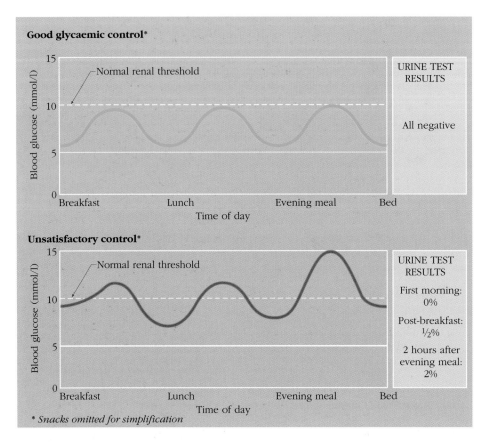

Figure 6.1 *Urine testing and the renal threshold for glucose.*

encompasses an education exercise. The following topics should be covered:

- why test?
- how and when to test
- which method of testing (with or without a meter)?
- the aims of testing (i.e. desirable blood glucose levels)
- how to adjust treatment (if the patient is willing and able to learn)
- when and where to seek help.

Guidelines for desirable results can be found on page 103.

Table 6.2 Urine testing strips currently available in the UK*

Trade name	Manufacturer	Test
Clinistix	Ames-Bayer	Glucose (limited range)
Diabur test 5000	Boehringer Mannheim	Glucose
Diastix	Ames-Bayer	Glucose
Ketodiastix	Ames-Bayer	Glucose + ketones

*In the UK, patients treated by diet alone, who are not entitled to free prescriptions, will find it less costly to purchase the test strips over the counter rather than on NHS prescription.

HBGM technique: HBGM involves obtaining a small blood sample by pricking the finger and applying a drop of blood to a test strip. An enzymic reaction takes place on the test strip pad, usually resulting in a colour change, which may be read either visually by matching the colour to a chart or electronically by placing the strip in a meter.

Table 6.3 The pros and cons of HBGM

Advantages	Disadvantages
■ Accurate blood glucose determination	■ Invasive procedure
■ Indicator of poor control	■ Fingers may become tender and painful
■ Indicator of hypoglycaemia	■ Needs to be carefully taught
■ Results facilitate adjustment of treatment	■ Inconvenient and time consuming
■ Increases patient's self-confidence	■ May cause anxiety when results are abnormal
	■ Inaccurate results when incorrectly performed
	■ Expensive

Using a meter generally improves the accuracy of the results, as both timing and reading are standardized. Certain meters incorporate special features, such as timing prompts or insufficient blood error prompts (Table 6.4). Unfortunately, meters have to be purchased by patients, and the cost may be prohibitive for some.

The technique of HBGM must be carefully taught by an experienced professional, such as a diabetes specialist nurse or a practice nurse. Obtaining the finger-prick blood sample may be painful if a needle or lancet alone is used. Special finger-pricking devices are available, making this process easier and less painful. Faulty technique, such as insufficient blood on the test strip, can produce inaccurate results; regular review of testing technique is essential.

When to test: In general, regular testing is best carried out before meals and before going to bed. If diabetes is stable and well controlled, testing once a day, but varying the time each day, will give an overall assessment of diabetic control. All results should be recorded in a diary as this allows trends in blood test results to be identified and treatment to be adjusted appropriately. More frequent testing will be necessary at times of poor control, adjustment of treatment, in pregnancy and during illness.

Some patients like to test their blood more frequently to enhance their sense of security. Frequent testing is invaluable when daily routine is erratic or vigorous exercise is undertaken.

Understanding the goals of treatment is a vital part of HBGM. Often patients become depressed because their blood glucose levels vary too much or it seems impossible to maintain levels within defined limits. It is important to explain to such patients the normal variability of glucose levels in diabetic patients and how sometimes results of tests are inexplicable. The main aim is to ensure the general trend of blood glucose levels is good and correlates with glycated haemoglobin values.

Table 6.4 Blood-testing strips and meters available in the UK

Test strip	Company	Type	Meter	Blood removal	Time
BM-Accutest	Boehringer Marnheim	Meter only	Accutrend	Non-wipe	12 seconds
BM-Test 1–44	Boehringer Marnheim	Visual or meter	Reflolux S	Wipe with cotton wool	120 seconds
Exactech	Medisense	Meter only*	Exactech[†]	Non-wipe	30 seconds
Glucostix	Ames-Bayer	Visual or meter	Glucometer GX	Blot with tissue	50 seconds
Glucotide	Ames-Bayer	Meter only	Glucometer 4[†]	Non-wipe	30–40 seconds
Hypocount	Hypoguard	Visual or meter	Supreme	Non-wipe	60 seconds
One Touch	Lifescan	Meter only	One Touch[†]	Non-wipe	45 seconds

*Meter does not read colour but measures the potential difference between two bars on the strip pad.
[†]Meter has an inadequate blood sample sensor.

Diabetes and travel

Diabetes should not be a barrier to travel for work or pleasure. Careful preparation is helpful, however, to ensure a smooth journey and an enjoyable trip.

The general practice team, who have up-to-date details of the recommendations concerning vaccinations and anti-malarial treatment, will be able to undertake appropriate immunization. Patients should also be advised to take a supply of codeine phosphate or loperamide for treatment of diarrhoea. It is useful to discuss with the patient how to manage diabetes during sickness and when to seek medical advice.

Insulin treated patients need reassuring that insulin can be kept at room temperature for about a month without undue deterioration, though if possible, it should not be left in direct sunlight or in a parked car in a hot country. Long journeys involving several changes of time zone may need special advice. An extra dose of short-acting insulin may be needed on long westward trips, omitting a dose or reducing doses for the eastward journey. Although glycaemic control may be upset by such changes, it generally settles within 1–2 days.

During the holiday season, diabetic patients should be asked whether they have particular holiday plans and the implications for their treatment discussed. The timing of meals often changes on holidays or business trips and more alcohol may be consumed, so patients need advice on management at such times. Holidays often involve a change in physical activity and, therefore, a change in treatment. Strenuous holidays, such as walking, cycling or skiing, generally need a 20% reduction in insulin or a lower dose of OHAs plus additional carbohydrate at meal and snack times. In hot countries, insulin may be absorbed more rapidly and appetite reduced. However, careful planning should enable patients to have a relaxed and enjoyable time.

Advice for diabetic patients travelling by air

- Preparation in the month before the flight:
  - obtain details of departure and arrival times
  - do not order special diabetic meals for the flight as they tend to be too low in carbohydrate
  - discuss adjustment of your treatment with your doctor or nurse
  - obtain a letter or card concerning your diabetes and its treatment to carry with you at all times
  - organize medical insurance for the trip.

- Packing for the flight:
  - pack an extra supply of carbohydrate in your hand baggage
  - pack insulin supplies in two separate pieces of hand baggage, as it may freeze in the hold and become inactive.

- During the flight:
  - soon after boarding, ask about timing of meals to help plan insulin treatment
  - if travelling alone, inform the stewardess that you have diabetes and are treated with insulin
  - select suitable food from in-flight meals and add extra carbohydrate from your own supply if necessary
  - avoid drinking excess alcohol
  - monitor blood glucose regularly (pre-meal or every 4–6 hours) and adjust insulin dose if necessary.

- On arrival:
  - adopt local time and meal times immediately even if this involves an extra dose of short-acting insulin
  - expect glycaemic control to be upset for a day or two following the journey and the time change.

Diabetes and employment

People with diabetes, particularly those treated with insulin, are considered ineligible for certain types of employment. In the UK, these include serving in the armed forces, flying as an airline pilot, working on offshore oil rigs and working in potentially dangerous conditions (e.g. deep sea diving). Certain services, such as the police or the fire service, do not recruit people with insulin treated diabetes, though subject to local variability, it may be possible for someone diagnosed after several years' service to retain their position.

General practitioners may be asked to provide a medical report concerning the suitability of a diabetic patient for a particular job. The assessment should be objective and should cover the patient's physical and mental capacity, standard of diabetic control (with reference to self-management and whether hypoglycaemia is a problem) and any complications that are liable to cause difficulties. If an objective assessment might harm the doctor–patient relationship, it is reasonable to ask a colleague or the local diabetologist to provide the required report.

Patient organizations can provide further information on employment for health care professionals, patients and employers (Figure 6.2)[1-3]. They may also be able to state their position on the employment of people with diabetes should anyone make an appeal concerning possible unjustified dismissal. In the UK, diabetic patients may be registered as disabled if they wish (though they seldom do) and this may be helpful for the purposes of training and job finding.

Medicolegal aspects of diabetes

Life insurance

People with diabetes are often upset when they are asked to pay higher insurance premiums than the non-diabetic population. Their anxiety and anger may be diffused by a simple explanation from an understanding health care professional.

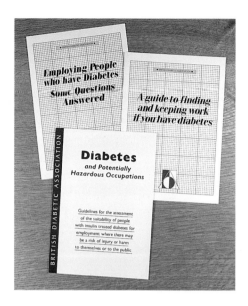

Figure 6.2 *Information from the British Diabetic Association for health care professionals, diabetic patients and potential employers on diabetes and employment.*

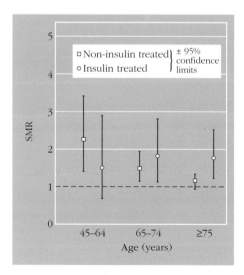

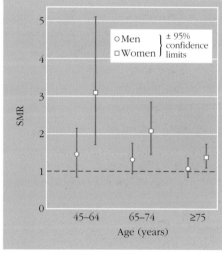

Figure 6.3 *Standardized mortality ratios (SMR) for all causes of death show the increased risk of premature death for diabetic patients[4].*
SMR = 1; no difference from the general population.

Insurance companies are not charities. The cost of the insurance premium is related to the degree of risk the insurance company takes when providing cover. People with diabetes are at greater risk of morbidity and mortality than non-diabetic people (Figure 6.3)[4]. Therefore, providing diabetic people with insurance cover demands a greater risk. To maintain solvency, the insurance company must balance this increased risk by an increased premium.

The premium a patient with diabetes might expect to pay may be up to two or three times that of the standard premium. Patients with diabetes are therefore advised to shop around insurance companies and seek the advice of an independent adviser. In certain circumstances, an insurance company may decline to offer cover to a particular diabetic client. In the UK, the British Diabetic Association (BDA) has an insurance service to help patients find suitable insurers.

Driving and motor insurance

When driving, people with diabetes are a potential hazard both to themselves and to the public, because of:

■ impaired mental functioning due to neuroglycopenia
■ complications of diabetes, which include poor visual acuity and cerebrovascular and ischaemic heart disease.

In Europe, drivers are required by law to declare their diabetes to the authorities. In the UK, the Driver and Vehicle Licensing Agency (DVLA) should be informed immediately diabetes is diagnosed or a driving licence is applied for, unless diet is the sole form of treatment. The DVLA must be notified if treatment is changed or if any complications develop. They must also be informed of gestational diabetes if insulin is required. Patients commencing insulin treatment are usually advised not to drive for a few days to avoid problems with unexpected hypoglycaemia.

Patients treated with insulin are allowed a restricted licence, renewable every 3 years, provided their condition is stable and a doctor responsible for their treatment signs a declaration that they are unlikely to be a danger on the road. Since 1991, insulin treated patients have been unable to acquire either a heavy goods vehicle or a public service vehicle licence. Drivers holding either of these licences before 1991 may be allowed to retain them, provided that they undergo an annual medical review by a consultant physician.

Some companies request higher motor insurance premiums from diabetic patients. It is worth asking a broker to obtain several quotes or to request information from a patient group, such as the BDA, who can obtain quotes for diabetic patients with no loading of the premium.

Driving licences are revoked in cases of the following complications:

■ loss of awareness of hypoglycaemia (see page 112 and page 262)

■ unstable diabetes (e.g. frequent episodes of hypoglycaemia or poor control)

■ visual complications (visual acuity must be better than 6/12 in one or both eyes and the visual field must be 120° width and at least 20° above and below the horizontal).

Doctors' responsibilities: physicians need to understand the legal requirements regarding driving so that they can educate their patients and assess their patients' driving capabilities.

Three key factors should be considered when assessing a patient's fitness to drive.

■ Is there evidence of cortical impairment such that the patient is likely to be a source of danger when driving?

■ Is the person liable to sudden and disabling episodes of altered awareness or loss of consciousness (e.g. due to hypoglycaemia in the absence of warning symptoms)?

■ Has the patient an adequate standard of vision (regarding both acuity and visual fields)?

If the patient fails in any of these areas, advice should be given (and recorded in the notes) to stop driving and to inform the licensing authorities and the motor insurance company.

Advice for diabetic patients: it is very important that patients are advised about driving either at diagnosis or when they reach legal driving age. The following points must be made clear.

■ The patient is responsible for informing the licensing authority and the relevant motor insurance company.

■ Patients should not drive if they experience any deterioration in eyesight and they should seek expert advice if night vision is affected.

■ Insulin treated patients and those taking a sulphonylurea should keep an emergency supply of quick-acting carbohydrate (e.g. glucose tablets; see page 109) in the vehicle. They should never drive having missed a meal or a snack and they should avoid driving for long periods without taking a rest for a meal.

■ Diabetic patients should always carry identification, including details of diagnosis and treatment, in case of a road traffic accident.

Shared care summary

Home monitoring

■ All patients should undertake home monitoring of diabetes on blood or urine samples. Testing techniques may be taught by either a diabetes nurse specialist or a practice nurse, who should review the patient's technique regularly.

■ Home monitoring should prove helpful to the patient in understanding diabetes, adjusting treatment and improving glycaemic control.

■ Patients need constant encouragement and motivation to carry out home monitoring.

Holidays and travel

■ Diabetes should not be a barrier to travel for business or pleasure.

■ Careful planning before a trip can help to avoid problems due to changes in activity, meals and time zones.

Employment and diabetes

■ People with diabetes, particularly those treated with insulin, are considered ineligible for certain types of employment (e.g. serving in the armed forces or flying airliners).

■ Family doctors may be asked to provide a medical report concerning the suitability of a diabetic patient for a particular job.

Insurance and driving

■ Doctors should explain to diabetic patients the legalities concerning declaration of their condition to licensing authorities and insurance companies.

■ Insulin-treated patients may qualify only for a renewable driving licence that is valid for a restricted period. In some countries, a patient is legally required to inform the licensing authorities of any change in treatment or complications.

■ Patients should be educated about sensible precautions to take when driving.

References

1 British Diabetic Association. *A guide to finding and keeping work if you have diabetes.* London: BDA, 1992.

2 British Diabetic Association. *Employing people who have diabetes: some questions answered.* London: BDA, 1992.

3 British Diabetic Association. *Diabetes and potentially hazardous occupations.* London: BDA, 1996.

4 Walters DP, Gatling W, Houston AC, Mullee MA, Julious SA, Hill RD. Mortality in diabetic subjects: an eleven-year follow-up of a community-based population. *Diabet Med* 1994; **11:** 968–73.

Further reading

Diamond Project Group on Social Issues. Global regulations on diabetics treated with insulin and their operation of commercial vehicles. *BMJ* 1993; **307:** 250–2.

Frier BM. Driving and diabetes. *BMJ* 1992; **305:** 1238–9.

Irvine R. The doctor, the driver and the law. *Practitioner* 1994; **238:** 668–70, 672, 674.

Lasch EM. The diabetic driver. *Diabetes Care* 1985; **8:** 189–90.

UK Driver and Vehicle Licensing Agency. *At a glance guide to the current medical standards of fitness to drive.* London: HMSO, 1993.

Chapter 7

Management of non-insulin dependent diabetes

Non-insulin dependent diabetes mellitus (NIDDM) is a common condition and its management is usually straightforward, though lifelong follow-up is required. NIDDM is an ideal candidate for the attentions of the primary health care team.

Serious long-term complications can be a major problem in patients with NIDDM, and are often present at diagnosis[1,2]. NIDDM certainly should never be considered a 'mild' form of diabetes (see pages 5 and 257).

This chapter focuses on maintaining near-normal blood glucose levels by diet, by therapy with oral hypoglycaemic agents (OHAs) or with insulin, and normalization of body mass index (BMI). Long-term follow-up is discussed in Chapter 11.

Goals of NIDDM therapy

The consensus on management of NIDDM has undergone a dramatic change. In the past, the main strategy was merely to treat primary osmotic symptoms, but the current approach includes trying to prevent or delay the onset of complications. Although the results of the Diabetes Control and Complications Trial (DCCT) may not be strictly applicable to NIDDM, other available evidence still suggests that those with constantly high blood glucose levels are more likely to develop complications. Definitive proof for this hypothesis may be forthcoming with the completion of the UK Prospective Diabetes Study (UKPDS). The UKPDS[3] is a 10-year study on 4500 patients with NIDDM randomized to different treatments.

In the general population, there is a well recognized association between hyperinsulinaemia and hyperlipidaemia, hypertension and cardiovascular diseases. There are theoretical concerns that intensifying pharmacological treatment for NIDDM, though diminishing risks of retinopathy, neuropathy and nephropathy, may conversely increase cardiovascular disease by causing hyperinsulinaemia. Firm evidence in support of this idea is lacking. It is essential, however, to monitor blood pressure and lipid levels while improving diabetes control with medication in NIDDM (Table 7.1). The aim should be to achieve glycaemic control within the good rather than the acceptable range. It is important, however, to minimize hypoglycaemia, so individual targets may require adjustment.

Initial assessment of the patient with NIDDM

A full assessment of the patient, including history, examination and investigations, is essential at diagnosis (Table 7.2). Home monitoring (usually urine testing) should be initiated and follow-up arranged. A typical management plan is outlined in Figure 7.1. The patient's details should also be added to the practice/district database register for NIDDM.

Reassurance during the consultation is vital. A simple explanation of the reasons for thirst and polyuria and the role of insulin may be followed by the reasons for altering eating patterns. During the clinical examination, it is important to inform the patient (though accompanied by reassurance) that the eyes, feet and heart are prone to damage as complications of diabetes and to advise on actions to avoid this damage. Any implications that this type of diabetes is 'mild' should be strictly avoided (see Chapter 1, page 5).

Referral to the hospital diabetes team

Occasionally, at presentation, patients with NIDDM are seriously ill and require hospital admission. Otherwise, in an ideal world, all newly diagnosed patients with NIDDM would be referred as

Table 7.1 European Consensus Guidelines for goals of therapy in NIDDM. Targets in the 'good' range are the ideal but may be unnecessary for certain patients (e.g. the elderly). Individual targets should be established for each patient. Reproduced with permission from the European NIDDM Policy Group[4]*

Metabolic targets	Good	Borderline	Poor
Blood glucose (mmol/l)			
Fasting	4.4–6.1	≤ 7.8	> 7.8
Postprandial	4.4–8.0	≤ 10	> 10
HbA$_{1C}$ (%)**	< 6.5	≤ 7.5	> 7.5
Total blood cholesterol (mmol/l)	< 5.2	< 6.5	> 6.5
HDL cholesterol (mmol/l)[†]	> 1.1	≥ 0.9	< 0.9
Fasting triglyceride (mmol/l)	< 1.7	< 2.2	> 2.2
BMI (kg/m^2)			
Men	< 25	≤ 27	> 27
Women	< 24	≤ 26	> 26
BP (mm Hg)	≤ 140/90[‡]	≤ 160/95	> 160/95

*For BDA targets used in the UK, see page 137.
Caution: reference ranges vary greatly depending on the method, so check local reference ranges. 'Good' is up to 3 SD above the upper limit of the mean value for the reference range (see page 137 for adjustment of targets according to local laboratory reference range).
[†]Target values for women are 0.3 mmol/l higher. If HDL cholesterol ≥ 1.7 mmol/l, LDL cholesterol should be calculated and more relaxed targets set for total cholesterol if the LDL cholesterol:HDL cholesterol ratio < 5.0 (most likely in postmenopausal women).
[‡]Stricter targets may be necessary in younger patients with early nephropathy.

Table 7.2 Initial assessment of a patient with newly diagnosed NIDDM

History

■ Current symptoms (including weight loss)
■ Current medication (withdraw thiazide diuretics, and steroids if possible)
■ Smoking history
■ Alcohol intake
■ Previous illnesses
■ Family history of diabetes
■ Symptoms related to complications:
  – cardiovascular (chest pain, dyspnoea, ankle swelling)
  – neurological (numbness, leg pain, impotence)
  – peripheral vascular (claudication, rest pain)
  – retinopathy (visual disturbance)

Examination

■ Measure height and weight; calculate BMI
■ Visual acuity, pupil dilatation and fundoscopy
■ Blood pressure
■ Heart and chest
■ Peripheral pulses
■ Abdomen for hepatomegaly (due to fatty liver)
■ Neurological examination of legs
■ Foot examination (for foot deformity or ulceration)

Investigations

■ Urine (glucose, protein, ketones)
■ Mid-stream urine (culture and sensitivity)
■ Plasma glucose and HbA_{1C}
■ Serum creatinine
■ Liver function tests
■ ECG (if cardiac history)
■ Fasting blood lipid profile after 3 months' stabilization of blood glucose

outpatients to the department of diabetes at the local hospital for assessment and advice. In certain areas, resources may be limited or the distance to the hospital too great for this to be practicable. A well-organized primary care team should have no difficulty in assessing, educating and managing newly diagnosed patients. In regions in which dedicated diabetes education programmes are available, patients should be referred unless there are either personal or sound medical reasons against this. Patients benefit from education by expert teachers and from the opportunity to meet other people with newly diagnosed diabetes. Definite criteria for specialist referral include:

- evidence of complications at diagnosis
- young women with NIDDM who are considering future pregnancies
- significant macrovascular disease requiring further investigation
- failure to gain good glycaemic control.

Dietary management of NIDDM

First aid dietary advice (Figure 7.2) should be given at the initial consultation with the aim of removing the primary symptoms of thirst and polyuria. In the longer term, overweight patients need to achieve weight reduction; target BMIs are given in Table 7.1. This commonly brings about a marked improvement in blood glucose. Motivation, weight monitoring and the practical aspects of devising weight reducing healthy diets have been considered in Chapter 5. All diabetic patients benefit from seeing a trained dietitian. In some, particularly elderly or frail patients with reduced life expectancy, dietary management may be relatively relaxed.

Physical activity

NIDDM tends to occur in middle-age or later when people are not involved in regular physical activity. Exercise promotes weight loss and also exerts favourable effects on blood glucose and lipid profiles, so it is to be recommended. Patients are often reluctant to accept the need for increased physical activity, so primary health care workers

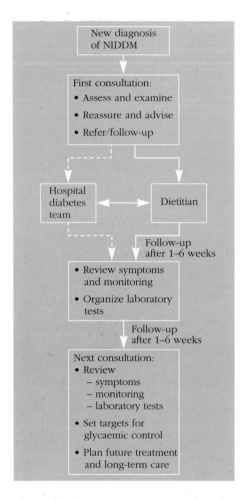

Figure 7.1 *Management of patients with newly diagnosed NIDDM.*

must be prepared to devote time for patient-centred counselling on this issue. Successful promotion of increased physical activity may be particularly difficult among members of certain cultural groups. For example, Asian women may object to swimming in public.

Treatment with OHAs

For the majority of patients, a trial of diet alone should continue for at least 4–6 weeks and, if progress is satisfactory, for 3 months. Patients with significant symptoms that are unresponsive to diet may need the introduction of an OHA earlier than this. Those presenting at diagnosis with a high blood glucose level (i.e. > 20 mmol/l) should be reviewed weekly for a few weeks to assess progress (see page 253). The magnitude of the initial blood glucose level does not always indicate the need for an OHA, as some patients ease their thirst with sugary drinks prior to diagnosis. In these patients, dietary measures alone may produce significant symptom relief and lowering of blood glucose.

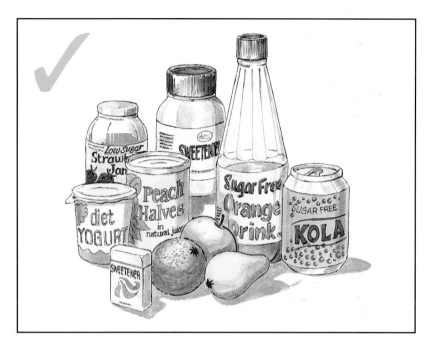

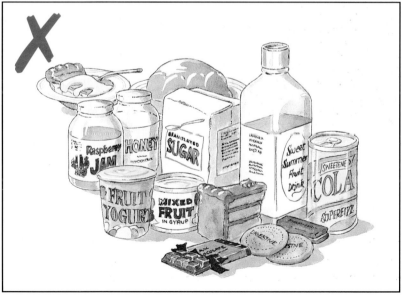

Figure 7.2 *First aid dietary advice for patients with NIDDM: avoid foods and drinks with added sugar.*

Types of OHA

There are three principal categories of OHAs (Table 7.3).

Sulphonylureas, most commonly prescribed to non-obese patients, act by:
■ increasing the sensitivity of pancreatic β-cells to glucose
■ increasing insulin secretion
■ reducing hepatic basal glucose output
■ enhancing the action of insulin on glucose uptake in muscle and other target tissues.

The net effect of these actions is to lower the blood glucose level, though weight gain is an undesirable side-effect. Hypoglycaemia may be induced (Table 7.4), particularly with the longer acting preparations (e.g. glibenclamide, chlorpropamide: see page 252); those with a shorter half-life (e.g. glipizide and gliclazide) carry less risk of hypoglycaemia[6]. Chlorpropamide and glibenclamide should be avoided in patients over 70 years of age or with renal impairment. Tolbutamide is a less potent and consequently, a less effective sulphonylurea than some of the newer agents.

Changing the prescription to an alternative sulphonylurea is not beneficial and it is never worth prescribing two to be taken in combination. All patients treated with sulphonylureas should be asked about hypoglycaemia, and those with frequent (more than once a week) or severe episodes should have their treatment reviewed. Hypoglycaemic symptoms mid-morning or before lunch are not uncommon. The dose of sulphonylurea may need to be reduced. Alternatively, patients who eat only a small breakfast or who are physically active in the morning may benefit from taking the sulphonylurea before their evening meal, particularly if this is the main meal of the day. Adjustment of diet (e.g. increasing the mid-morning snack) can help to reduce hypoglycaemia but may promote weight gain.

Table 7.3 OHAs currently in use

	Renal impairment	Liver disease	Drug interactions
Sulphonylurea			
■ glibenclamide	Avoid	Avoid any sulphonylurea or use in small doses only	Alcohol, cimetidine, corticosteroids, fibrates, fluconazole, miconazole, NSAIDs, phenothiazines, sulphonamide, trimethoprim
■ gliclazide	Caution*		
■ glipizide	Caution*		
■ gliquidone	Caution*		
■ tolazamide	Caution*		
■ tolbutamide	Caution*		
■ chlorpropamide	Avoid		
Biguanide			
■ metformin	Avoid in renal failure	Avoid	Alcohol, cimetidine[5]
α-glucosidase inhibitor			
■ acarbose	Avoid in moderate to severe renal failure	Avoid	Cholestyramine, pancreatin

*Increased risk of hypoglycaemia.

Biguanides have several postulated modes of action:

■ inhibition of hepatic gluconeogenesis
■ enhancement of insulin action on peripheral tissues
■ reduction of gastrointestinal glucose absorption.

Metformin, the only biguanide currently available, should be used as first-line therapy in obese patients following dietary trial. It may be used successfully in combination with a sulphonylurea. Metformin is contraindicated in patients with advanced heart failure. Its use is limited by its tendency to cause gastrointestinal upset (Table 7.4), which can be minimized by taking the tablets after food and only gradually increasing the dose. It is best to commence metformin at a dose of 500 mg b.d. Intermittent diarrhoea is a dose-dependent side-effect that is more common with higher doses, so some patients manage with a dose reduction.

Table 7.4 Side-effects of OHAs

Side-effect	Sulphonylureas	Metformin	Acarbose
Hypoglycaemia	+*	–	–
Drug interaction	+	+	–
Hypersensitivity	+	–	–
Gastrointestinal upset	–	+	+
Lactic acidosis	–	+	–
Hyponatraemia	+	–	–
Cholestasis	+	–	–
Malabsorption of folate, vitamin B_{12}	–	+	–
Hyperinsulinaemia	+	–	–
Weight gain	+	–	–

*Particularly with longer acting preparations.

α-**glucosidase inhibitors** provide a different approach to treatment – inhibiting the digestive enzymes responsible for the hydrolysis of sucrose and starch with the release of glucose. When these enzymes are inhibited, the sucrose and starch pass further down the intestinal tract for later hydrolysis and absorption. The overall effect is a delayed and reduced postprandial blood glucose peak. The α-glucosidase inhibitor, acarbose, has been used extensively in Europe either as monotherapy or as an adjunct to treatment by diet and other OHAs when glycaemic control remains unsatisfactory.

A comparative study showed a similar improvement in blood glucose and glycated haemoglobin levels with acarbose, 100 mg t.d.s., or glibenclamide, 4 mg (mean daily dose), suggesting a considerable difference in potency between acarbose and sulphonylureas[7]. However, acarbose leads to a significant reduction in postprandial insulin levels compared with glibenclamide.

When taken as monotherapy, acarbose does not cause hypoglycaemia, but when used in conjunction with other agents, hypoglycaemia cannot be treated with sucrose or complex carbohydrate, as their hydrolysis will be limited. Systemic side-effects are unlikely with acarbose, as at therapeutic doses, less than 2% of the agent is absorbed, but gastrointestinal effects, such as flatulence, abdominal distention, diarrhoea and borborygmus, commonly occur (Table 7.4). These effects may be reduced by the gradual introduction of the drug, starting at 50 mg once or twice daily, and slowly increasing over 2–3 months.

Adjusting OHAs

It is wise for primary care physicians to limit the use of OHAs to a small number with which they are familiar. Sulphonylureas generally lower blood glucose levels more than biguanide or acarbose therapy. The dose response to sulphonylureas tends to tail off with increasing dose. Consequently, the first tablet has a much greater effect than increasing the dose from three to four tablets, probably because the

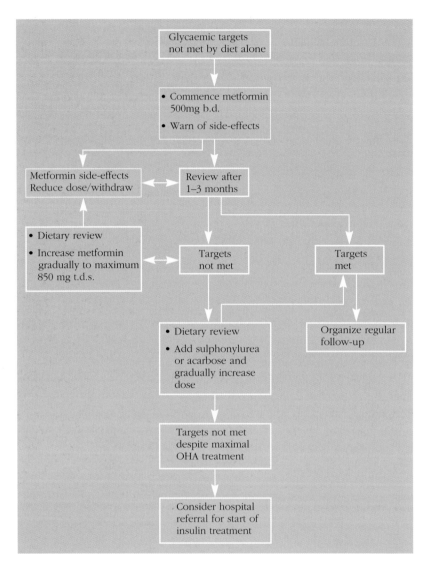

Figure 7.3 *Initiating OHAs in obese patients with NIDDM. See Table 7.1 for glycaemic targets.*

remaining pancreatic β-cells are already being maximally stimulated. Thus, it is often disappointing when increasing to the maximal dose of a sulphonylurea to see only a minimal improvement in blood glucose levels.

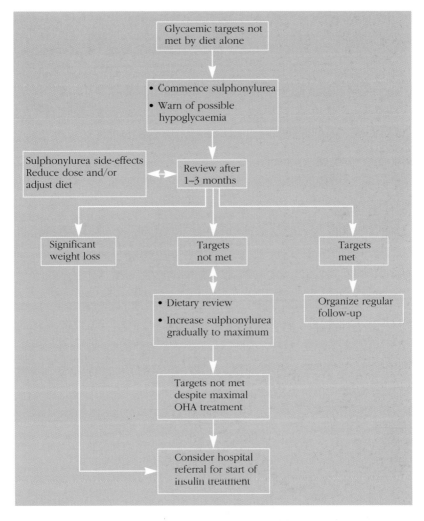

Figure 7.4 *Initiating OHAs in non-obese patients with NIDDM. See Table 7.1 for glycaemic targets.*

Combination treatment may be valuable, and certainly, metformin may be helpful in limiting the weight gain often seen with sulphonylureas (Figure 7.3). For those patients who are underweight and are poorly controlled despite maximal sulphonylurea therapy, adding in metformin is seldom appropriate. A switch to insulin therapy is advisable in most cases (Figure 7.4).

87

Results from the UKPDS show that the natural history of NIDDM involves gradually deteriorating glycaemic control despite dietary and OHA treatment (see page 272). It is likely, therefore, that following initial stabilization, additional therapy will be required over the years. When introduction of insulin therapy is contemplated, it should not be postponed, as long periods of poor control increase the risk of developing complications.

Other treatment options

Glycaemic control has been improved in overweight patients with NIDDM by anorectic agents[8]. These agents may act by stimulating serotoninergic pathways and consequently stimulating the satiety centre in the brain. Dexfenfluramine is an appetite suppressant whose use had led to improved diabetic control, though it may be taken for only 3 months. Fluoxetine is an antidepressant that improves glycaemic control through weight loss. It may also improve the patient's mood and increase motivation.

A small improvement in blood glucose levels is also seen when using fibrates to treat hyperlipidaemia (see page 191).

Insulin therapy

A significant proportion of patients with NIDDM require insulin therapy at some stage. The most common reason for conversion to insulin therapy is failure to achieve adequate glycaemic control. The cause of this lack of control is usually progressive β-cell failure. In addition, patients with NIDDM, who are otherwise well controlled, may require insulin during acute illness, for treatment of hyperosmolar coma, during surgical procedures, or even for treatment of specific diabetic complications, such as painful neuropathy or amyotrophy. Pregnancy is another indication for insulin treatment, which is best commenced before a planned pregnancy.

Starting insulin therapy should not be delayed even in the elderly, despite concerns about hypoglycaemia or injection technique. If necessary, insulin may be introduced on a trial basis with specific criteria agreed between physician and patient. All patients converted to insulin therapy require education (see Chapters 4 and 8), frequent monitoring and supervision (e.g. in the community by a diabetes specialist nurse) during the first few weeks.

Shared care summary

■ NIDDM is usually diagnosed in primary care.

■ At diagnosis, the patient should be given a simple explanation and reassured by the GP. A full assessment should be undertaken, looking particularly for evidence of complications, which may already be present.

■ First aid dietary advice should be explained at diagnosis by the primary care team. Subsequently all patients require assessment and education by a dietitian.

■ Patients with NIDDM are usually treated by diet alone for at least 4–6 weeks before adding OHAs if glycaemic control remains unsatisfactory. Patients should be warned of side-effects of OHAs.

■ Patients not well controlled by maximal doses of OHAs should be referred to the hospital diabetes team.

■ Insulin treatment should be considered early. Patients starting insulin should be reviewed by the hospital diabetes team and insulin started with supervision by a diabetes nurse specialist.

■ Patients with complications or considering pregnancy should be referred to the hospital diabetes team.

■ Patients with NIDDM require long-term follow-up, which may be undertaken in primary or secondary care or in a shared care programme.

References

1 UK Prospective Diabetes Study. 6. Complications in newly-diagnosed type 2 diabetic patients and their association with different clinical and biochemical risk factors. *Diabetes Res* 1990; **13:** 1–11.

2 Harris MI. Noninsulin-dependent diabetes mellitus in black and white Americans. *Diabetes Metab Rev* 1990; **6:** 71–90.

3 The United Kingdom Prospective Diabetes Study. 13. Relative efficacy of randomly allocated diet, sulphonylurea, insulin, or metformin in patients with newly diagnosed non-insulin dependent diabetes followed for 3 years. *BMJ* 1995; **310:** 83–8.

4 European NIDDM Policy Group. *A desktop guide for the management of non-insulin dependent diabetes mellitus (NIDDM). 2nd edn.* Brussels: International Diabetes Federation, 1993: 8.

5 Monson JP. Selected side-effects: II. Metformin and lactic acidosis. *Prescribers J* 1993; **33:** 170–3.

6 Anon. Oral hypoglycaemics for diabetes. When and which? *Drug Ther Bull* 1991; **29:** 13–16.

7 Hoffman J, Spengler M. Efficacy of 24-week monotherapy with acarbose, glibenclamide or placebo in NIDDM. The Essen study. *Diabetes Care* 1994; **17:** 561–6.

8 Rachman J, Turner RC. Drugs on the horizon for treatment of type 2 diabetes. *Diabet Med* 1995; **12:** 467–78.

Further reading

Joint Working Party of the British Diabetic Association, the Research Unit of the Royal College of Physicians and the Royal College of General Practitioners. Guidelines for good practice in the diagnosis and treatment of non-insulin dependent diabetes mellitus. *J R Coll Physicians Lond* 1993; **27:** 259–66.

Hadden D. Managing the newly diagnosed maturity-onset patient. In: Tattersall RB, Gale EAM eds. *Diabetes clinical management.* Edinburgh: Churchill Livingstone, 1990: 39–56.

Watkins PJ, Drury P, Taylor K. *Diabetes and its management.* Oxford: Blackwell Scientific Publications, 1990.

Chapter 8

Management of insulin treated diabetes

This chapter deals with the management of all insulin treated patients – those with ketosis prone insulin dependent diabetes mellitus (IDDM) and those with non-insulin dependent diabetes mellitus (NIDDM) requiring insulin for effective blood glucose control. All patients requiring insulin treatment should be referred to the diabetologist for advice and the diabetes nurse specialist for education and support. However, many practices are now taking on the long-term follow-up of these patients or operating a shared care policy.

Self care, though relevant to all diabetic patients, is of paramount importance to those treated with insulin. Today, all diabetic patients are encouraged to enjoy as normal a lifestyle as possible; diabetes should not be allowed to dominate life. However, certain basic principles (consistent insulin administration, careful monitoring and regular food intake) must be followed if diabetes is to be controlled. Problems are generally encountered when these principles are ignored. Organization, discipline and a good memory are all necessary for effective diabetes management. Few people can boast that they consistently display all these qualities, so it is not surprising that patients with diabetes have problems from time to time.

Types of insulin

Although a large number of different insulin preparations are available, they may be classified simply in three main categories:

short-acting insulin; long- or intermediate-acting insulin; and very long-acting insulin (Figure 8.1). The manufacturers' data sheets suggest subtle differences in duration of action between products within each category. These are unimportant in clinical practice and patients tend to have individual responses to different insulin preparations.

Since the advent of genetic engineering, it has been possible to produce human insulin in large quantities using genetically programmed bacteria. Some patients need reassurance that human insulin is not derived from human sources. Current patient anxieties over human insulin are considered in Chapter 9 (page 114). As human insulin tends to act slightly more quickly and cause less antibody production, a small dose reduction is wise on transfer from animal to human insulin.

Insulin administration, absorption and action

Insulin administration

With modern fine needles, insulin injections are virtually painless. Patients who have a needle phobia require special help and support. They may use special injectors or pens that have no exposed needle.

Insulin may be taken by syringe, pen device or pump. Many patients use special plastic disposable syringes calibrated in insulin units and with fixed needles. It is common practice to use the same syringe until the needle is blunt or injections become painful (usually after 2–7 days). Subcutaneous infections associated with injection sites are seldom seen and are usually due to factors such as poor diabetic control.

The new insulin pen devices (Figure 8.2) simplify insulin administration, as the required dose is simply 'dialled up' on the pen before injection. The majority of patients started on insulin now use an insulin pen. Certain types of pen may be repeatedly reloaded with a new cartridge of insulin and used for years, while others are

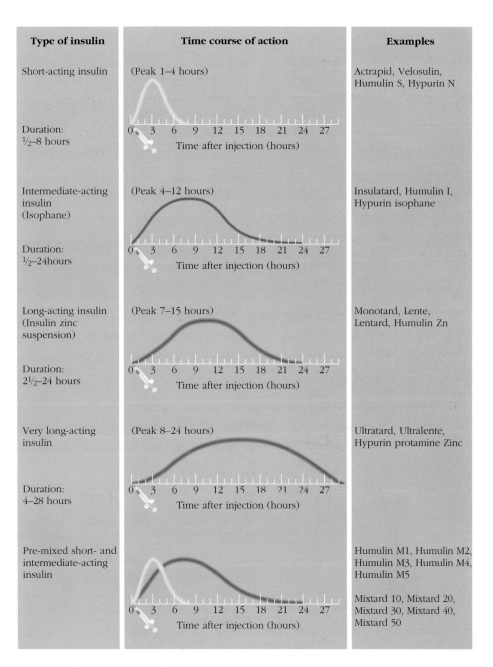

Figure 8.1 *Time course of action for various insulin preparations following subcutaneous injection at time zero.*

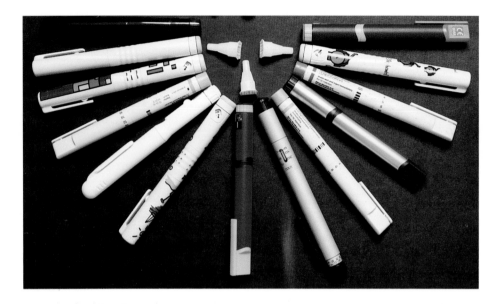

Figure 8.2 *Insulin pen devices.*

preloaded and disposed of when the cartridge is empty. Although insulin pens are relatively straightforward, patients need careful training in their use (Figure 8.3). The pens have proved robust and reliable and are conveniently carried in the pocket or handbag.

Insulin may be continuously supplied by an insulin pump but since the advent of insulin pens, there is little advantage in this method. In general, insulin pumps are expensive. Their use is not widespread and should be supervised by the hospital diabetes team.

Injection sites and insulin absorption
Generally, insulin should be taken approximately 15–30 minutes before a meal, except for the recently introduced insulin lispro (see page 244). Patients should be encouraged to vary their injection sites, as repeated injection into the same area inevitably leads to tissue damage and scarring (Figure 8.4). This in turn tends to alter the rate of insulin absorption and may lead to erratic control and unexpected hypoglycaemic attacks. Insulin is absorbed most quickly from the

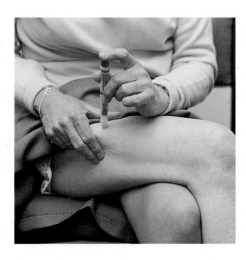

Figure 8.3 *Insulin injection technique with a pen device.*

abdomen and most slowly from the thighs and buttocks; the arms are intermediate[1]. Any factors affecting the blood supply to the injection site (e.g. physical activity, hot weather or a hot bath) will affect the rate of absorption. The volume of insulin solution injected (i.e. the total dose) also affects the absorption rate, as smaller volumes have a greater surface area to volume ratio and hence are absorbed faster. It should be borne in mind that slower absorption means a longer duration of action. Mixing long- and short-acting insulins, which is quite acceptable, may alter the predicted duration of insulin action. As the clearance of insulin is prolonged in renal failure, dose reduction is necessary.

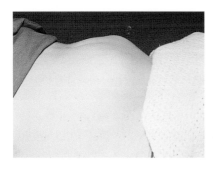

Figure 8.4 *Abdominal lipohypertrophy resulting from repeated insulin injection.*

Insulin regimens (Figure 8.5)

Once-daily insulin: a single daily injection of a long-acting insulin taken before breakfast in the morning is a most unreliable and unsatisfactory method of controlling diabetes. The slow rise in insulin level during the morning fails to control the post-breakfast glucose peak. The insulin level rises as the day progresses giving rise to hypoglycaemia during the evening or night. The duration of action is usually less than 24 hours, and fasting glucose levels are high. The use of this regimen to keep injections to a minimum in elderly patients should be abandoned.

A single dose of long-acting insulin taken before bedtime has been used to treat patients with NIDDM who fail to respond to maximal doses of oral hypoglycaemic agents (OHAs). This corrects the fasting hyperglycaemia and allows residual insulin secretion stimulated by OHAs to deal with the postprandial glucose peaks. Hypoglycaemia may be avoided by careful insulin dose adjustment.

Twice-daily insulin is the most commonly used insulin regimen. Insulin injections are given before breakfast and before the evening meal, usually as a mixture of short- and long- or intermediate-acting insulins, such as Actrapid plus Monotard or Velosulin plus Insulatard. The proportions used are generally one-third short-acting to two-thirds long-acting. Premixed insulins (Figure 8.1) simplify the administration, and a wide range of these is available.

Some patients (e.g. those with some endogenous insulin secretion or those physically active patients who suffer from pre-lunch hypoglycaemia with the usual mixed regimen) are managed better with twice-daily intermediate-acting insulin (usually an isophane preparation).

Three-times-daily insulin: nocturnal hypoglycaemia at 2–4 a.m. is a common problem for patients taking twice-daily short- and long-acting insulin. The long-acting insulin peaks early in the night and then tends to run out before the morning. These patients benefit from splitting the evening dose of insulin, taking the short-acting

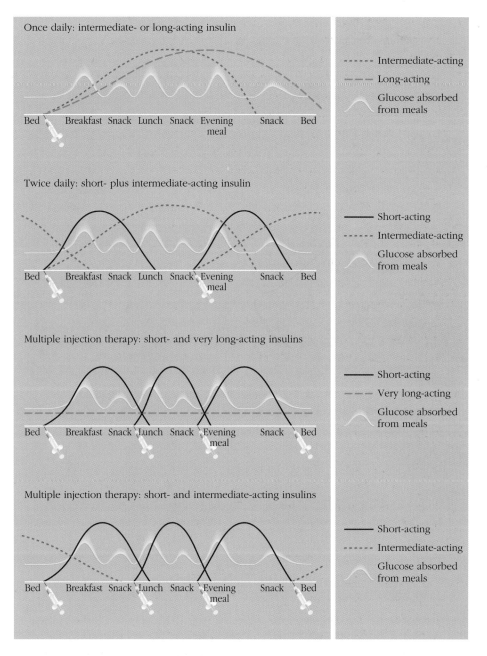

Figure 8.5 *Various types of insulin regimens.*

insulin as usual before the evening meal and the long-acting component just before retiring to bed. It is not necessary to eat after taking the long-acting insulin, as it will not be absorbed for several hours. However, a late evening snack is recommended for all insulin treated diabetic patients.

Insulin four times a day or multiple injection therapy (MIT): short-acting insulin is taken before each meal and long- or very long-acting insulin is taken at bedtime. An insulin pen is usually used for the preprandial doses to simplify insulin administration. The bedtime insulin can be given by pen (if isophane) or syringe (if Monotard or Ultratard, which are not available in pen cartridges). This regimen has the advantage of flexibility, as meal timing is less critical. Dose adjustments may be made if exercise or eating patterns vary. For optimal control, this regimen requires a high level of motivation and a good memory, as missed insulin doses cause significant problems. If this regimen is used to achieve tight glycaemic control, hypoglycaemic episodes may occur more frequently unless regular snacks and meals are eaten. The new insulin analogue, lispro (see page 244), may be advantageous in this situation.

Patients using the very long-acting preparations (e.g. Ultratard) have a permanent background level of insulin, and this may contribute to hypoglycaemia, particularly in mid-afternoon. Another significant drawback of the very long-acting preparations is the time lag in response to dose adjustments; it takes 2–3 days before the effect of a dose change is seen. This is frustrating when rapid adjustment is necessary (e.g. in response to illness or nocturnal hypoglycaemia).

Choosing an appropriate insulin regimen

It is most important to choose the right regimen for each patient. Although insulin treatment is for life, the regimen does not have to be. Physicians should be prepared to be flexible and respond to changes in the patient's lifestyle and understanding. The most appropriate regimen is the one with which the patient feels most comfortable.

At diagnosis, an assessment can be made of the usual lifestyle, including work patterns (e.g. shift work, extensive travel) and hobbies, particularly sporting activities. Other factors include the patient's personality, cultural background, intellect and ability to cope. Although it is best to start with the optimal regimen, the shock of diagnosis may render the patient temporarily incapable of taking on anything but the most simple method of treatment.

Choice of insulin treatment in people with NIDDM follows the same principles, but although insulin treatment in an obese patient with poorly controlled NIDDM often makes the patient feel better, it inevitably leads to weight gain. Careful attention to diet is imperative, and certain patients benefit from continuing metformin with their insulin treatment. It may keep weight gain to a minimum while increasing insulin sensitivity, thereby allowing the use of smaller doses of insulin (see page 271).

When glycaemic control is unsatisfactory in insulin treated patients, the tendency to opt for a 'quick fix' by switching to MIT should be considered carefully. The results of such a change may be disappointing if the fundamental reason for poor control, which may be lack of motivation or dietary indiscretions, has neither been appreciated nor addressed. Control may deteriorate even further as the patient struggles with an unfamiliar regimen.

Starting insulin treatment

These days, relatively few patients present with ketoacidosis requiring hospital admission. All newly diagnosed patients with IDDM should be referred to hospital the same day. Children always require urgent referral, but adult patients (provided they are not dehydrated) may be referred during usual working hours to the diabetes specialist by telephone or fax. All hospital diabetologists should have a system whereby newly diagnosed patients can be seen within 1 or 2 working days.

Many centres commence insulin treatment without admitting the patient to hospital. Initial education of the patient is taken on by the diabetes nurse specialist, who may visit the patient at home and provide continuing support during this difficult period. Subsequent education, which needs to cover many aspects of life (see Chapter 4), may be organized at the local diabetes centre, carried out by the hospital diabetes team or supplemented by the primary health care team, particularly the district nurse, who may be involved with initial home care. Conversion of patients with NIDDM to insulin can similarly be undertaken at home and closely supervised by the diabetes nurse specialist and district nurse.

When treatment is commenced on an outpatient basis, a small dose of insulin is initially used and gradually increased over the following few days according to the results of home blood glucose monitoring (HBGM). Stabilizing the diabetes and elucidating the optimal insulin dose may take several weeks and good overall control (as assessed by glycated haemoglobin; see page 13) may not be achieved for several months.

Diabetic patients who are blind or only partially sighted require special attention to manage their insulin administration and diabetes. Many are independent in daily living and are reluctant to rely on someone else for the insulin injections. Giving the injection is not a problem, but drawing up the correct dose can be. The new disposable insulin pens can be managed by many poorly sighted patients giving them total independence rather than relying on a relative or a district nurse to leave loaded syringes in the refrigerator.

Dietary management of insulin treated diabetes

All insulin treated patients should be assessed and advised by the dietitian at diagnosis. They normally require several sessions, which are best carried out over several weeks. Periodic review during the first year is also necessary to check progress and adjust dietary intake in the light of changes in weight. Thereafter, formal dietary review should be undertaken at least every 2–5 years, depending on the patient.

Patients treated with insulin need to eat carbohydrate-containing foods at regular intervals throughout the day in order to reduce the risk of hypoglycaemia. Unfortunately, current insulin regimens do not reflect normal physiology. From subcutaneous injection, insulin levels are slow to rise and continue to peak for a considerable time (Figure 8.5) predisposing to hypoglycaemia. Thus, even with MIT, the short-acting insulin (except for insulin lispro – see page 244) does not rise rapidly enough to prevent significant postprandial glucose peaks and unless a snack is eaten 2–3 hours after injecting, hypoglycaemia is likely to occur before the next meal. The consumption of slowly digested high-fibre carbohydrate is valuable in reducing postprandial glucose peaks and prolonging glucose absorption.

The usual method of coping with the required regular food intake is to have three meals plus three snacks spread through the day. Sometimes, two snacks are needed if the time between main meals is prolonged. It is not surprising that many diabetic people regard eating as a chore rather than a pleasure. Suggesting interesting foods (particularly low-fat snacks) is an important role for the dietitian (see page 52).

Optimizing glycaemic control

In the past, patients were not encouraged to adjust insulin doses, and many are still anxious about doing so. Attitudes have changed, however, and patients may now be given advice on adjusting their own insulin doses (Table 8.1). Patients need to work closely with their doctors or nurses as they take on insulin adjustment. The most important principle is that adjustments should not be made too frequently. It is always wise to wait until it is possible to see a pattern developing over a few days rather than adjusting on a daily basis. One possible exception is adjustment of short-acting insulin by patients on MIT, though even these patients should not begin making adjustments until they are familiar and experienced with the regimen.

In theory, adjusting insulin doses to gain good control throughout the day should be straightforward, provided that the insulin regimen is understood (i.e. which insulin dose is acting when; Figure 8.5). In practice, insulin adjustment is not so simple because the insulin dose is not the only factor affecting the blood glucose level. Other factors include food intake, timing of food, timing and site of insulin injection

Table 8.1 Patient guidelines for adjusting insulin treatment to improve glycaemic control

■ Adjust only one dose of insulin at a time.

■ Wait at least 3 days to observe effects of a dose change.

■ Make only small adjustments in insulin dose: dose 1–10 units, adjust by 1–2 units at a time; dose 11–39 units, adjust by 2 units at a time; dose > 40 units, adjust by 4 units at a time.

■ First adjust insulin or dietary intake to avoid recurring episodes of hypoglycaemia.

■ Second, adjust evening long-acting dose of insulin so that first morning glucose lies between 4 and 7 mmol/l with no hypoglycaemia during the night.

■ Next, adjust morning fast-acting insulin dose if hypoglycaemia becomes a problem before lunch.

■ Finally, adjust daytime insulin doses gradually to obtain overall good control.

■ Expect glucose control to improve over a period of weeks rather than days.

and exercise. Other issues may also complicate the picture (e.g. a common cold, a woman's menstrual cycle, stress levels). The aim should be to gain good control overall and certainly not to expect all HBGM results to be good. Guidelines for glucose results in patients treated with insulin are presented in Table 8.2.

First adjustments of insulin should be to correct problems of recurrent hypoglycaemia, which will help to win the patient's confidence. The next step is to obtain good fasting glucose levels by adjusting the evening long-acting insulin dose. The morning short-acting dose may then need reducing or the mid-morning snack increasing.

Table 8.2 Guidelines for blood glucose objectives for patients treated with insulin

Ideal targets

- Preprandial blood glucose: 4–7 mmol/l
- Pre-bedtime blood glucose: 6–8 mmol/l
- Two-hour postprandial blood glucose: < 10 mmol/l
- Mild hypoglycaemic episodes, kept to a minimum
- No severe hypoglycaemic episodes

In practice these targets may be difficult to achieve; they should be adjusted for individual patients.

In some cases, increasing night-time insulin doses leads to hypoglycaemia during the night. This may require a change in regimen, such as a switch to three times a day (see page 96). Patients must understand that a bedtime snack (though *not* a large takeaway meal) is seldom the reason for high morning blood glucose. Blood glucose levels rise overnight when there is insufficient insulin in the body to stop the liver from producing glucose.

Once fasting glucose levels lie in the correct range, attention may be shifted to other results during the day, focusing initially (if appropriate) on the second long-acting insulin dose and the glucose results during its duration of action. Final adjustments are in the short-acting insulin doses.

A common error when patients adjust their own insulin doses is to alter the bedtime long-acting insulin dose according to the pre-bedtime blood glucose. This is inappropriate as the pre-bedtime blood glucose relates to the evening short-acting dose and the food taken. The long-acting dose needs to be adjusted according to fasting blood glucose and in relation to any night-time hypoglycaemic attacks.

Some patients demonstrate very erratic HBGM results with no clear pattern. The cause may be multifactorial. Sometimes it is due to varying food intake, eating quickly absorbed carbohydrate, erratic meal times or overreaction to hypoglycaemic attacks. Different degrees of physical activity on different days or too frequent adjustment of insulin doses are other common reasons.

Shared care summary

■ On diagnosis, patients with IDDM require assessment and advice on management. Education and support are provided by the hospital based diabetes nurse specialist but may also involve the primary care team.

■ Patients with NIDDM, whose glycaemic control is inadequate with maximal doses of OHAs, should be referred to the hospital diabetes team for assessment and transfer to insulin therapy.

■ All insulin treated patients need dietary assessment and education by a dietitian when starting insulin and at regular intervals during follow-up.

■ The hospital diabetes team need to supervise the patient during the initial period of stabilization with insulin treatment (usually about 6 months).

■ Lifetime follow-up can be successfully shared between the primary and secondary care teams.

Reference

1 Henriksen JE, Djurhuus MS, Vaag A. Impact of injection sites for soluble insulin on glycaemic control in Type 1 (insulin-dependent) diabetic patients treated with a multiple insulin injection regimen. *Diabetologia* 1993; **36:** 752–8.

Further reading

Insulin therapy in diabetes. An interactive, computerized education programme produced by Lilly Diabetes Care in association with Medicomp Software. Further information from: Lilly Diabetes Care, Dexter Court, Chapel Hill, Basingstoke RG2 5SY. Tel: (01256) 315000.

Chapter 9

Hypoglycaemia: prevention and treatment

For insulin treated diabetic patients, hypoglycaemia is a major source of anxiety, which for many overshadows any fears of the complications of diabetes. For the health care professional, understanding the position of hypoglycaemia in the patient's priorities is essential for successful diabetes management.

This chapter describes the clinical picture of hypoglycaemia, its manifestations and its reversal. The problem of asymptomatic hypoglycaemia or hypoglycaemia unawareness is also considered in the light of recent research. Hypoglycaemic coma is considered in more detail in the next chapter on diabetic emergencies.

Clinical picture of hypoglycaemia

Hypoglycaemia arises when the blood glucose concentration falls below normal physiological levels.

Physiological responses to hypoglycaemia

The normal response to an undue fall in blood glucose is the release of various hormones, including adrenaline, glucagon and cortisol. This response leads to replenishment of glucose both from glycogen stores and from gluconeogenesis. Adrenaline release and the characteristic symptoms of hypoglycaemia (see below), which are driven by the sympathetic nervous system, occur in healthy human volunteers at a blood glucose concentration of about 3.6 mmol/l (Figure 9.1). A continued fall below 3 mmol/l results in cerebral

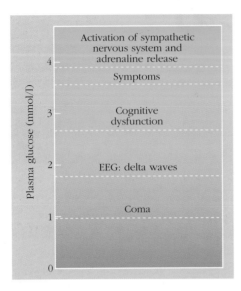

Figure 9.1 *Physiological responses to hypoglycaemia in non-diabetic volunteers.*

dysfunction, which is manifest as an inability to think clearly or to carry out simple everyday actions. Confusion and drowsiness are evident at levels below 2 mmol/l and coma below 1 mmol/l. If the blood glucose pool is not replenished (due either to the inbuilt hormonal mechanism or to treatment), the coma proves fatal. Profound hypoglycaemia is often accompanied by fitting, which causes hypoxia and exacerbates the effects of the cerebral glucose deficit.

Since in non-diabetic people, pathological hypoglycaemia requiring investigation (e.g. for an insulinoma) is defined as a blood glucose concentration below 2.8 mmol/l, the necessity for diabetic patients to avoid blood glucose levels of less than 4 mmol/l has not been fully appreciated by medical professionals[1]. Recent research (see below) has emphasized the need for a change in professional attitudes, with modification of patient education and monitoring targets.

Symptoms of acute hypoglycaemia

Common symptoms of acute hypoglycaemia are listed in Table 9.1. The symptoms actually experienced vary with the individual but tend

Table 9.1 Typical symptoms of acute hypoglycaemia

Autonomic	Neuroglycopenic	General
Tremor	Dizziness	Hunger
Feeling hot	Confusion	Weakness
Sweating	Tiredness	Blurred vision
Anxiety	Difficulty speaking	Drowsiness
Nausea	Inability to concentrate	Shivering
Palpitations	Headache	
	Visual disturbance	

to be repetitive within one patient for a given set of circumstances. Patients learn to recognize their own symptom pattern and to take corrective action. Problems tend to occur when the symptom pattern changes or recognition is delayed (e.g. when very tired or after alcohol consumption).

Close friends or relatives often notice subtle changes in the diabetic patient (Table 9.2) that warn of impending hypoglycaemia; the patient may then be prompted to eat, though such prompting may be a source of friction in the relationship. It is imperative that all patients with insulin dependent diabetes mellitus (IDDM), or with non-insulin dependent diabetes mellitus (NIDDM) treated with a sulphonylurea (see page 82), alert their friends and colleagues to the symptoms of hypoglycaemia.

A small number of insulin treated patients experience hypoglycaemic symptoms when the blood glucose is still in the normoglycaemic range. Control in these patients is generally very poor, with blood glucose levels generally above 10 mmol/l. Under these circumstances, the glucose sensor in the brain that detects hypoglycaemia (see page 112) adapts to the higher level of glucose. These patients need understanding and encouragement to improve their glycaemic control gradually over a period of weeks or months.

Table 9.2 Other presentations of hypoglycaemia

- Personality changes (e.g. unusually irritable or tearful)
- Mood changes (e.g. becoming depressed and negative)
- Behavioural changes (e.g. showing atypical/'primitive' behaviour, becoming unduly aggressive, performing odd actions, behaving as if under the influence of alcohol)
- Development of focal neurological deficit (e.g. hemiparesis, dysphasia)
- Maintenance of 'automatic' behaviour
- Loss of consciousness or impossible to arouse from sleep
- Unusually disturbed sleep
- Excessive nocturnal sweating
- Fitting

The glucose sensor will then revert to a response at truly hypoglycaemic levels.

Treatment of hypoglycaemia

All diabetic patients treated with insulin or sulphonylureas should be warned about the symptoms of hypoglycaemia and educated in its management. Treatment of hypoglycaemia is composed of three essential elements.

- The blood glucose level should be raised as quickly as possible by eating quick-acting carbohydrate (Figure 9.2).

- The blood glucose should be prevented from falling subsequently by eating slowly absorbed carbohydrate (Figure 9.2), which is **in addition to normal snacks and meals.**

- The reason for the hypoglycaemic attack should be identified so that another attack in similar circumstances may be avoided in the future.

Generally speaking, unless the trigger is vigorous exercise, about 20 g carbohydrate should be sufficient to treat an attack of

First, quick-acting carbohydrate

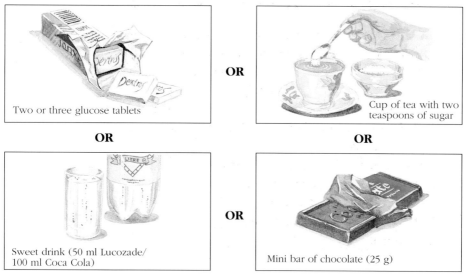

Two or three glucose tablets

OR

Cup of tea with two teaspoons of sugar

OR

OR

Sweet drink (50 ml Lucozade/ 100 ml Coca Cola)

OR

Mini bar of chocolate (25 g)

Follow with 10–20 g slow-acting carbohydrate

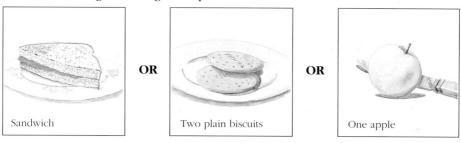

Sandwich

OR

Two plain biscuits

OR

One apple

Figure 9.2 *Carbohydrate foods and drinks for treatment of hypoglycaemia.*

hypoglycaemia, but patience is of the essence. It may take 10–15 minutes for the symptoms to subside.

Once the hypoglycaemic episode has been successfully treated, the patient should continue with the usual insulin regimen. Patients (or health care professionals) may suggest a delay or a reduction in the following insulin dose, but this is inappropriate and tends to cause high blood glucose levels later in the day.

Identifying the cause of a hypoglycaemic episode is just as important as treating the event (Table 9.3). Frequent hypoglycaemic attacks require reappraisal of the entire diabetes management plan, including diet and insulin regimen, monitoring and patient education. Elucidating the reason for attacks is sometimes difficult. Delayed hypoglycaemia, which often occurs during the evening or the night, is particularly puzzling for patients. It often follows an unusual day involving vigorous activity. Although extra carbohydrate has been consumed at the time, it may have been sufficient to avoid hypoglycaemia but insufficient to cover the exercise. Afterwards, when the muscles are subsequently recharging their glycogen stores, this process may cause hypoglycaemia.

Prevention of hypoglycaemia

More frequent hypoglycaemic attacks seem to be an inevitable consequence of striving towards tighter glycaemic control. Indeed, the Diabetes Control and Complications Trial showed a 2–6-fold increase

Table 9.3 Checklist to investigate the cause of a hypoglycaemic attack

- Check carbohydrate intake. Any missed meal or snack?
- Any increase in exercise? Was sufficient extra carbohydrate taken?
- Review injection sites. Delayed absorption can occur from lumpy areas (lipohypertrophy).
- Review insulin dose or sulphonylurea treatment.
- Discuss alcohol consumption, as alcohol reduces awareness of hypoglycaemia and inhibits gluconeogenesis.
- Consider role of menstrual cycle. Insulin requirements may fall on day 1.
- Was hot weather or a hot bath the cause? Either would accelerate insulin absorption.

in the incidence of serious hypoglycaemia when patients were switched to intensive insulin therapy[2]. The majority of hypoglycaemic episodes are avoidable with the following precautions:

■ complete understanding by the patient of the causes of hypoglycaemia
■ complete understanding by the patient of strategies to avoid hypoglycaemia
■ no delay or omission of meals or snacks
■ a sensible diet with plenty of unrefined carbohydrate to promote slower digestion and glucose absorption
■ accurate and correct insulin doses
■ avoidance of large additional insulin doses to correct high blood glucose levels
■ maintenance of full carbohydrate diet even if the blood glucose is high
■ consumption of extra carbohydrate if activity is increased
■ adjustment of insulin doses when vigorous or prolonged activity is planned
■ constant maintenance of a ready supply of glucose tablets/sweets and prompt action at the earliest warning symptoms.

Frequency of hypoglycaemic attacks

The majority of insulin treated patients experience some hypoglycaemic episodes, but serious attacks (see page 119) need to be avoided. Patients with pronounced warning symptoms may be prepared to have one or two mild episodes a week, but those with poor warning symptoms (see below) need to avoid even these. Patients tend to forget or deny hypoglycaemic episodes, so it is difficult to obtain an accurate picture of the frequency of attacks without resorting to questioning partners or carers[3]. Most patients when questioned believe they are being asked about serious hypoglycaemic attacks, but in fact it is important to find out about mild attacks as well. Careful questioning may elicit surprising answers. It is inadvisable for any patient to have frequent, even if only mild, hypoglycaemic episodes.

Loss of warning symptoms of hypoglycaemia

Clinical problem of asymptomatic hypoglycaemia

Loss of the symptoms of impending hypoglycaemia means that the first warnings of hypoglycaemia are neuroglycopenic symptoms typical of cerebral dysfunction. The patient is then unable to interpret or react to the problem. Patients with this problem of asymptomatic hypoglycaemia are in danger of severe hypoglycaemic attacks with loss of consciousness, fitting, brain damage and death.

Although this problem *may* occur soon after diagnosis, its prevalence tends to increase with increasing duration of diabetes. About one-third of patients with IDDM for over 15 years report loss of warning symptoms[4]. Those at greatest risk are those who have already had an attack of severe hypoglycaemia and those being treated intensively with the aim of achieving near normoglycaemia.

Although it is the autonomic warning symptoms that are delayed, this problem is not caused by autonomic neuropathy[4]. Animal work has shown that the sensor in the brain that is responsible for detecting hypoglycaemia and triggering the counterregulatory response, may be affected by hypoglycaemic episodes. In non-diabetic volunteers, the threshold at which the hormonal and symptomatic response to hypoglycaemia occurred was lowered by a previous episode of hypoglycaemia[5]. In insulin treated diabetic patients, the threshold for triggering the response to hypoglycaemia may fall to quite low levels of glucose (e.g. less than 2.5 mmol/l). Consequently, when the hormonal and symptomatic response occurs, there is already cerebral dysfunction and cognitive impairment (i.e. the early warning symptoms of hypoglycaemia have been lost). This fall in the threshold has been shown following the introduction of multiple injection therapy (MIT; see page 97; Figure 9.3)[6].

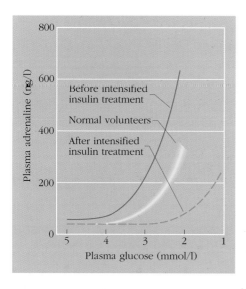

Figure 9.3 *Adrenaline response to induced controlled hypoglycaemia in patients with IDDM before and after 6 months of intensified insulin therapy[6].*

Reversibility of asymptomatic hypoglycaemia

It has been postulated that the adaptive change in the cerebral glucose sensor might be reversible. Accordingly, studies were undertaken with patients suffering from asymptomatic hypoglycaemia either treated with MIT or with conventional insulin therapy. Diabetes management was adjusted until no hypoglycaemic episodes were experienced. After 3 weeks' stabilization without hypoglycaemia, it was possible to demonstrate in the laboratory a significant improvement in the hormonal response to hypoglycaemia — from 2.4 mmol/l to 3.4 mmol/l, at which level the symptomatic responses once more preceded cerebral dysfunction (Figure 9.4)[1]. Therefore, it is feasible to help patients to regain their warning symptoms. Moreover, in this study, despite the avoidance of hypoglycaemia, overall glycaemic control as judged by glycated haemoglobin did not change.

Strategies to help patients with asymptomatic hypoglycaemia

All patients who experience asymptomatic hypoglycaemia should be referred to the hospital diabetes team. It is vital to try and explain the problem of asymptomatic hypoglycaemia to patients and to try to

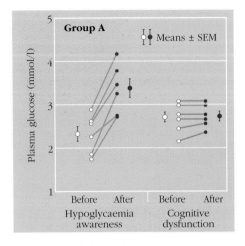
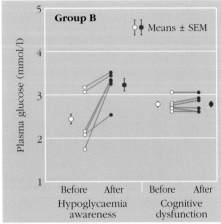

Figure 9.4 *Reversibility of asymptomatic hypoglycaemia. Plasma glucose levels at which subjects first became aware of hypoglycaemia before and after a 3-week period of scrupulous hypoglycaemia avoidance. Group A were patients with well controlled diabetes and Group B poorly controlled. Reproduced with permission from Amiel SA[1].*

motivate them to work with you to overcome it. The importance to the patient of avoiding even mild episodes of hypoglycaemia cannot be overemphasized. The entire management plan requires review in order to avoid hypoglycaemic episodes completely (Table 9.4). An absence of regular carbohydrate consumption and reluctance to take regular snacks are common problems, so motivation and frequent monitoring are vital.

Human insulin and current patient anxieties

Over the last few years, considerable controversy has arisen concerning human insulin and whether it has played a role in the loss of warning symptoms of hypoglycaemia. Unbalanced reporting by the media has fuelled anxiety among patients (see page 262). Human insulin has been blamed for various problems with little scientific evidence.

Human insulin is absorbed slightly more quickly than animal insulins and tends to have a shorter duration of action. Careful

Table 9.4 Strategies to help patients with asymptomatic hypoglycaemia

- Immediate action to avoid future hypoglycaemic attacks
- Advise partner/relatives/friends/workmates how to treat hypoglycaemia
- Organize dietary review, particularly type and distribution of carbohydrate
- Ensure regular snacks between meals and before bedtime
- Examine insulin injection sites and avoid areas of lipohypertrophy or atrophy
- Review insulin regimen in light of work and activities
- Review insulin doses and proportions of long- and short-acting insulin
- Discuss insulin adjustment and avoid too frequent or too large adjustments
- Review home blood glucose monitoring technique and equipment
- Discuss frequency and timing of monitoring
- Check blood glucose at 2 a.m. when adjusting regimen and insulin doses
- Review management of exercise
- Consider safety to drive/operate machinery/undertake certain types of work
- Counsel on openness regarding diabetes diagnosis

double-blind studies in which neither the patient nor the doctor knew which insulin species was being investigated, have shown no evidence that human insulin is more likely than pork insulin to cause asymptomatic hypoglycaemia. However, there is a group of patients who claim that following a switch to human insulin, they lost their symptomatic warnings of hypoglycaemia. Many of these patients report that returning to pork insulin restored these warning symptoms.

Personal observation suggests that these patients still have problems with lack of hypoglycaemia awareness, but some patients generally feel more comfortable taking animal insulin. If a patient requests a return to animal insulin, it is wise for the doctor to agree to the transfer. At the same time, careful attention should be paid to the underlying causes of the hypoglycaemic attacks (see page 110). For some reason, this particular anxiety about human insulin appears to be confined mainly to the UK.

Shared care summary

■ All patients treated either with a sulphonylurea or with insulin should be warned about hypoglycaemia and the symptoms to expect.

■ They should be taught how to treat hypoglycaemia and how to prevent it.

■ Patients should be asked about hypoglycaemic episodes at each clinic visit.

■ Severe episodes of hypoglycaemia are usually treated by family practitioners, who should investigate the cause of the attack.

■ All patients with asymptomatic hypoglycaemia should be referred to the hospital for assessment, advice and treatment.

■ Insulin treated patients may regain early warning symptoms of hypoglycaemia by adjustment of treatment to avoid hypoglycaemic episodes.

References

1 Amiel SA. RD Lawrence lecture 1994. Limits of normality: the mechanisms of hypoglycaemia unawareness. *Diabet Med* 1994; **11:** 918–24.

2 The DCCT Research Group. Epidemiology of severe hypoglycaemia in the Diabetes Control and Complications Trial. *Am J Med* 1991; **90:** 450–9.

3 Heller S, Chapman J, McCloud J, Ward J. Unreliability of reports of hypoglycaemia by diabetic patients. *BMJ* 1995; **310:** 440.

4 Hepburn DA, Patrick AW, Eadington DW, Ewing DJ, Frier BM. Unawareness of hypoglycaemia in insulin-treated diabetic patients. Prevalence and relationship to autonomic neuropathy. *Diabet Med* 1990; **7:** 711–17.

5 Heller SR, Cryer PE. Reduced neuroendocrine and symptomatic responses to subsequent hypoglycaemia after 1 episode of hypoglycaemia in nondiabetic humans. *Diabetes* 1991; **40:** 223–6.

6 Amiel SA, Sherwin RS, Simonson DC, Tamborlane MV. Effect of intensive insulin therapy on glycemic thresholds for counterregulatory hormone release. *Diabetes* 1988; **37:** 901–7.

Chapter 10

Avoiding and treating diabetic emergencies

Although one of the main aims of diabetes management is to educate patients and health professionals to avoid problems, emergency situations do occasionally arise and they require rapid medical action. In this chapter, three types of coma that may occur in uncontrolled diabetes are considered. The problem of steroid treatment in diabetic patients is also discussed.

Hypoglycaemic coma

The prevention and treatment of mild-to-moderate hypoglycaemia has been covered in Chapter 9. However, if prompt action is not taken, the blood glucose level may continue to fall causing coma as the brain receives inadequate glucose for normal function. This type of coma develops rapidly over a matter of minutes, often during the night and particularly in patients who no longer experience adequate warning symptoms (see page 112). It is commonly caused by inadequate food intake (e.g. a missed meal or snack) or insufficient food for the physical activity performed.

Hypoglycaemia should be considered as the most likely cause of sudden loss of consciousness in a diabetic patient treated with insulin or a sulphonylurea. A finger-prick blood glucose estimation can confirm the diagnosis. If hypoglycaemia is excluded, other causes may then be considered (e.g. a cardiovascular accident, a drug overdose, a head injury, etc.).

Treatment of hypoglycaemic coma

If the patient is semiconscious, with a gag reflex present, oral carbohydrate may be administered. This needs to be a sugary drink followed, once the patient is more aroused, by more slowly digested carbohydrate (e.g. biscuit, small sandwich). If the patient is unconscious, 1 mg glucagon should be administered subcutaneously and Hypostop® gel may be squirted around the lips. These may be given by a relative or friend. Glucagon takes 15 minutes to raise the blood glucose. If the patient does not return to consciousness within 15 minutes, intravenous glucose is necessary and a doctor must be called. In the UK, ambulance paramedical staff are also trained to give glucagon and treat hypoglycaemic coma.

When called to a patient in a hypoglycaemic coma, it is important to carry out the following procedure.

■ Ensure that the patient has a patent airway and give oxygen if cyanosed.

■ Give an intravenous injection of 25–50 ml of 50% dextrose solution, which usually restores consciousness immediately, or subcutaneous glucagon, 1 mg. If relatives have already given glucagon, do not give another dose of glucagon but instead, use intravenous glucose. Glucagon will be ineffective if liver glycogen stores are low.

■ When consciousness is restored, make sure that the patient eats a snack containing 20–30 g carbohydrate.

■ Check that the patient has not been injured while unconscious, particularly if fitting occurred, and that brain function is normal.

■ Investigate the cause of the hypoglycaemic attack and discuss with the patient and relatives or friends how a similar attack may be avoided in future.

■ Discuss with partner, family or friends whether they would be willing to give glucagon, and prescribe it. Advise them to use the dextrose gel, Hypostop®, on future occasions, provided that the patient is still semiconscious.

Following a hypoglycaemic coma, the patient may remain confused for some time. If there is no improvement in consciousness with 50 ml of 50% glucose, either the diagnosis is incorrect or the patient has suffered significant brain damage. In either case, immediate transfer to hospital is necessary. Patients suffering from hypoglycaemia secondary to sulphonylurea treatment also require hospital admission, as hypoglycaemia can be recurrent and prolonged.

Hyperglycaemic comas

Hyperglycaemic comas, whether diabetic ketoacidosis (DKA) or hyperosmolar non-ketotic coma (HONK), are due to absolute or relative insulin deficiency, which often arises during intercurrent illness.

Acute intercurrent illness in diabetic patients

Like the rest of the population, patients with diabetes contract infections, such as colds, gastroenteritis, urinary tract infections, etc. Any type of illness generally upsets diabetic control causing blood glucose levels to rise. This is due to the release of hormones, such as cortisol and adrenaline, which help the body to cope with the illness. These hormones antagonize insulin action, rendering it less effective. More insulin than usual is required to counteract this. Patients need educating about managing their diabetes during these illnesses (see panel overleaf). A common error is to stop taking insulin or tablets (in anticipation of hypoglycaemia) when the appetite is poor or vomiting is a problem. The resulting insulin deficiency leads to high blood glucose levels and, if unchecked, DKA or HONK.

Another mistake is to take frequent doses of syrupy cough linctuses, which elevate the blood glucose even further. Many sugar-free linctuses are now available either with or without a prescription (Table 10.1, page 123).

DKA

DKA usually develops less dramatically than hypoglycaemia. The symptoms gradually worsen over a period of hours or 1–2 days. The pathways contributing to ketoacidosis are outlined in Figure 10.1

Sick-day rules

Coughs, colds, 'flu', gastric 'flu' and food poisoning need prompt attention, as they usually increase the need for insulin. If you are ill:

1 **Never stop, or even reduce, your insulin dose.**
2 Measure blood glucose more frequently (e.g. four times a day; before breakfast, before lunch, before the evening meal and at bedtime).
3 If blood glucose remains below 11 mmol/l, continue with your normal insulin dose.
4 If blood glucose is above 11 mmol/l, consider dose adjustment and discuss with your medical adviser or the diabetes team.
5 If you are unable to eat, replace your normal carbohydrate with milk or a glucose drink (such as Lucozade® or a fruit cordial). Drink plenty of sugar-free fluids (at least 5 pints (3 l)/day).
6 If you have a temperature, take two paracetamol or two aspirin tablets up to four times a day.
7 If your blood glucose is over 17 mmol/l, if you are vomiting and cannot keep down liquids, if you are alone, or if you do not know what to do, it is essential to contact your doctor or a member of the diabetes team.

(page 124). Ketoacidosis may induce nausea and vomiting, further exacerbating the metabolic disturbance. Hyperventilation, triggered by acidosis, causes even further dehydration.

Early recognition of the signs and symptoms of hyperglycaemia and appropriate adjustment of treatment means that DKA can be avoided. Indeed, the incidence of DKA is lower than in the past, thanks to increased awareness among family physicians and better patient education. When the patient has any of the problems listed in Table 10.2 (page 125), hospital referral should be considered. It is preferable to admit patients to hospital at an early stage before severe DKA develops.

Table 10.1 Sugar-free linctuses for common coughs

Non-prescription linctus	Prescribable linctus
Benylin — Children's Cough Linctus	Galenphol
Bronalin Junior Linctus	Pavacol-D
Covonia for children	
Dimotane Co	
Dimotane Co Paediatric	
Expulin Cough Linctus	
Expulin Dry Cough Linctus	
Expulin Children's Cough Linctus	
Meltus Baby Linctus	
Meltus Dry Cough Elixir	
Meltus Junior Dry Cough Elixir	

Treatment of DKA: Patients with established DKA should be transferred to hospital. If there is evidence of shock (tachycardia, poor peripheral perfusion and hypotension), intravenous fluids should be started immediately with 500 ml of plasma expander, followed by 0.9% saline. Speedy transfer to hospital is important.

HONK

Non-ketotic coma, in which there is hyperglycaemia and severe dehydration, is just as dangerous as DKA. Indeed, the mortality risk is greater, particularly for the elderly and those with other serious illnesses.

The primary cause of HONK is relative insulin deficiency, which leads to hyperglycaemia, osmotic diuresis, dehydration, loss of electrolytes and circulatory failure (Figure 10.2). Ketoacidosis does not occur because the small amount of circulating insulin that is present in patients with non-insulin dependent diabetes mellitus (NIDDM) inhibits ketogenesis.

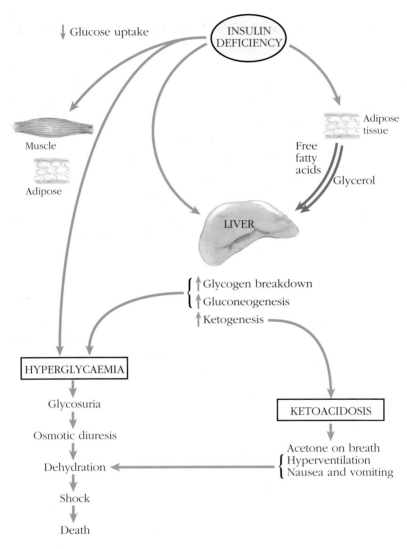

Figure 10.1 *Mechanism of metabolic disturbances in diabetic ketoacidosis.*

HONK is not easily diagnosed but should be considered in patients with NIDDM treated with tablets or diet. Risk factors for HONK are listed in Table 10.3. A substantial proportion of patients with HONK

Table 10.2 Indications for hospital referral in a diabetic patient

- Persistent vomiting for more than 4 hours
- Signs of dehydration
- Any disturbance of consciousness
- Hyperventilation
- Inability to take adequate oral fluids
- Significant ketonuria (more than a trace on dip-stick testing)
- Acute illness in pregnancy
- Suspected myocardial infarction
- Stroke
- Trauma

are subsequently found to have previously undiagnosed diabetes. Non-specific deterioration in general health over a period of days is common, possibly with associated confusion. On examination, patients are very dehydrated, but they do not hyperventilate. The severe dehydration often leads to thrombotic complications, particularly cerebral, and mortality is high. Any patient suspected of having HONK should be urgently admitted to hospital.

Differential diagnosis of diabetic comas

Although the differential diagnosis of impaired consciousness in diabetes may be problematic in the home, there are several distinguishing features, and diagnosis is easy if a good history is available from a friend or relative. The sweet smell of acetone on the breath is an immediate pointer to DKA, provided that the physician is capable of detecting it. A finger-prick blood test will immediately indicate hypo- or hyperglycaemia. A urinary glucose test is unreliable and may be misleading, whereas heavy ketonuria is a strong indicator of DKA. Dilated pupils are common in hypoglycaemia, as is a drenching sweat. Hyperventilation and vomiting are both indicators of metabolic

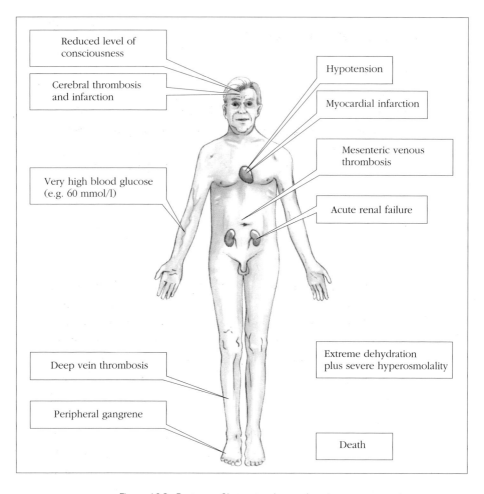

Figure 10.2 *Features of hyperosmolar non-ketotic coma.*

acidosis, and signs of dehydration also indicate a hyperglycaemic coma. In the absence of any of these signs, a cerebrovascular event or even self-poisoning should be borne in mind.

Diabetes management during steroid therapy

Diabetes is not a contraindication to the use of steroids for treatment of medical conditions, such as asthma, temporal arteritis, etc.

Table 10.3 Risk factors for HONK

- Old age
- Infection
- Antihypertensive medication (e.g. diuretics)
- Consumption of large quantities of glucose-containing drinks (e.g. Lucozade®)
- Race (e.g. more common in West Indian patients than in Caucasians)
- Undiagnosed diabetes
- Poorly controlled NIDDM

Deterioration in glycaemic control is likely to occur, however, on initiation of steroid therapy. Patients should be warned appropriately.

When steroids are first introduced, the patient should monitor diabetes more closely. As steroids usually have their effect within a week, the patient should be reviewed at this stage. Small doses (at most 5 mg prednisolone daily) may require little change in diabetes treatment. A short, reducing course of steroids for asthma may only temporarily upset control.

Steroids are generally given at higher dosage and for longer periods of time. Patients taking oral hypoglycaemic agents (OHAs) may require transfer to insulin treatment, while those already taking insulin require larger doses. A once-daily dose of prednisolone typically causes high blood glucose in the evening, which improves by the following morning. Multiple injection therapy is usually necessary for good control of diabetes while taking steroids. Diabetic patients treated with steroids should be referred to the hospital specialist for assessment and advice on further management.

When the steroid dose is reduced or withdrawn, the insulin dose should be decreased. Insulin requirements before the steroid treatment was instituted may be used as a guide.

Shared care summary

■ The family practitioner is most likely to be called out to a diabetic patient with impaired consciousness.

■ Differential diagnosis relies on a history from attendant family or friends and signs, such as excessive sweating and dilated pupils (hypoglycaemia), or acetone on the breath and hyperventilation (DKA), or dehydration (HONK).

■ If a finger-prick blood test confirms hypoglycaemia, immediate treatment with intravenous glucose, 20–50 ml of 50% solution, or subcutaneous glucagon, 1 mg, is essential and should restore consciousness. If these methods fail, the patient should be transferred to hospital immediately.

■ When restored to consciousness, the patient should eat a snack containing approximately 20 g slowly absorbed carbohydrate.

■ Investigation of the cause of hypoglycaemia is important in order to avoid a repeat episode.

■ Immediate hospital referral is essential for any patient with signs of HONK or DKA.

■ Steroid therapy disturbs glycaemic control, so patients given steroids should be warned to monitor blood glucose closely. Those with deteriorating glycaemic control should be referred to hospital for assessment and management advice. Transfer to insulin treatment may be necessary.

Further reading

Bolli GB, Gale EAM. Hypoglycaemia. In: Alberti KGMM, Defronzo RA, Keen H, Zimmet P eds. *International textbook of diabetes mellitus.* Chichester: John Wiley & Sons, 1992: 1131–50.

Tattersall RB, Gale EAM. Hypoglycaemia. In: Tattershall RB, Gale EAM eds. *Diabetes clinical management.* Edinburgh: Churchill Livingstone, 1990: 228–40.

Chapter 11

Long-term follow-up

Chronic hyperglycaemia has profound metabolic consequences, which lead to tissue damage in many organs. Diabetic patients therefore have greater morbidity and a higher mortality rate than non-diabetic people due to the development of microvascular complications and macrovascular disease. As there is now clear evidence that good glycaemic control can delay the development of these complications, the aim of diabetes management must be to strive for as good glycaemic control as is possible within the constraints set by the dangers of hypoglycaemia and the patient's lifestyle and cultural characteristics. Thorough long-term follow-up involving motivation, monitoring of glycaemic control and prevention or early detection of complications is essential. Both primary and secondary care sectors are involved in this long-term follow-up.

In this chapter, the management principles outlined in Chapters 7 and 8 are extended to cover long-term care, which is essentially similar for both insulin dependent (IDDM) and non-insulin dependent (NIDDM) diabetes. Standard protocols for routine clinic visits and for the all-important annual review are presented.

Whose responsibility?

In the UK, the family practitioner has the responsibility for the medical needs of the patients on his/her list. If the family practitioner is unable to provide appropriate care, the patient is referred to a specialist. The new contract relating to chronic disease management reinforces this responsibility.

Table 11.1 Suggested protocol for performing an annual review

About 2 weeks before clinic appointment

Blood test for:
- glucose, glycated haemoglobin or fructosamine
- serum creatinine
- lipid profile (i.e. total cholesterol, triglyceride, high density lipoprotein cholesterol)

Early morning urine test for microalbuminuria

Day before clinic appointment

Patient notes collected and checked to see that all results are available

Clinic routine

- Measure weight and height; calculate body mass index
- Test urine for glucose, ketones and protein; send mid-stream urine to laboratory if protein present
- Ask about general health and any problems
- Ask about symptoms of vascular diseases (e.g. angina, dyspnoea, claudication) and discuss laboratory lipid results with patient
- Ask about symptoms of neuropathy (e.g. numbness, paraesthesia, impotence)
- Ask about alcohol consumption and cigarette smoking
- Look at self monitoring results (urine or blood) and laboratory glucose/HbA_{1C}/fructosamine; inform patient of laboratory results and review and discuss glycaemic control
- Ask if any problems with control/insulin treatment the patient would like to discuss
- Measure blood pressure after 5 minutes' rest
- Measure distant visual acuity, dilate pupils with tropicamide, 1%, and perform fundoscopy; if eye screening is carried out elsewhere, arrange for this to be done prior to the clinic visit
- Examine feet for deformities, ulcers and infection; feel foot pulses; test vibration, light touch and reflexes

- Examine injection sites
- Carry out further clinical examination and/or organize further investigation as indicated
- Discuss findings with patient; encourage and agree targets for following year
- Organize referral to dietitian, chiropodist, specialist nurse, consultant diabetologist, ophthalmologist as appropriate
- Complete patient record card/cooperation booklet and patient notes
- Arrange next appointment and update computer system if appropriate

The patient should be involved in the choice of long-term follow-up. Certain patients should always be referred to the hospital for follow-up and these include:

- all children and adolescents
- all women who are pregnant or considering pregnancy
- all patients with significant complications or unusual problems.

Follow-up for the remaining patients depends on the expertise available in the practice. In some areas, patients with NIDDM are followed in general practice while those with IDDM are followed at the hospital diabetes clinic. Other districts operate a shared care system with all patients attending the hospital clinic annually. Each practice must agree the approach to their patients' follow-up with the local diabetes department. This approach must ensure high quality care for all and must be flexible to allow patients to benefit from any advances in diabetes management.

Table 11.1 suggests a suitable protocol for an annual review, which may be carried out either in general practice or at the hospital clinic. Special problems arising between annual reviews may be dealt with initially in general practice, though referral may prove necessary. A standard protocol for routine clinic visits is suggested in Table 11.2.

Table 11.2 Suggested protocol for a routine visit to a diabetes clinic either in general practice or in a hospital outpatient department

About 2 weeks before clinic appointment

Blood test for glucose, HbA_{1c} or fructosamine

Day before clinic appointment

Patient notes collected and checked to ensure blood test result available

Clinic routine

- Weigh patient and compare weight with previous visit
- Test urine for glucose, ketones and protein
- Ask about general health and any problems since last visit
- Look at self monitoring results (urine or HBGM) and laboratory blood test; review glycaemic control and discuss with patient
- Agree targets for next visit with patient
- Review management of any identified complications or risk factors
- Perform examination or organize any necessary investigation
- Ask if the patient wishes to discuss anything
- Record details of visit in patient record card or cooperation booklet and in patient notes
- Arrange next appointment
- Update computer records if appropriate

Essential components of long-term care

People with diabetes have a lifelong illness requiring lifelong follow-up. An important component of care is development of the patient/doctor (or nurse) relationship. Patients should expect to see the same doctor or nurse at each clinic visit, allowing the relationship to flourish and promoting improved understanding of individual patient problems.

Encouragement of self care

The widespread recognition, particularly by doctors, of the patient's central role in diabetes care represents an important advance. Today, patients are encouraged to monitor their diabetes and to adjust treatment to optimize diabetic control. To undertake this potentially difficult role, patients require extensive education about diabetes and a willingness to learn from their own life experiences. With time, many acquire considerable skills and demonstrate remarkable insights into diabetes management.

Health care professionals in turn must adapt their roles and recognize the patients' expertise. Working *with* the patient should be the aim. A patient's ability for self care might at first sight appear poor because of high blood glucose or glycated haemoglobin results, but hasty judgements should be avoided, as diabetes is a highly variable disease. It should not be forgotten that the patient may have lived with diabetes for many years. The patient's agenda may not coincide with that of the health care professional. Addressing the patient's worries first may enable other issues to be tackled more successfully later.

Some patients are reluctant to embrace all aspects of care, though there is seldom complete rejection. Lack of acceptance of the diabetes diagnosis is a common problem. For these patients, denial may be a coping mechanism. Therefore, exhorting them to monitor their diabetes fails because it is asking them to recognize their diabetes. Such patients are often non-attenders at the clinic. If this problem of denial persists, it may be helpful to utilize counselling skills or to enlist the help of a psychologist. The health care worker may need to discuss these difficult cases with colleagues in order to cope with the inevitable feelings of anxiety and frustration. Modifying targets for glycaemic control is one approach that may be helpful in the pursuit of a good long-term working relationship with the patient.

Continuing education on all aspects of diabetes

Although newly diagnosed patients are usually educated about diabetes at the hospital, they may be overloaded with information at this time. Repetition and reinforcement are constantly required (see Chapter 4) and at each clinic visit, the patient's knowledge should be assessed. It may be a good idea to cover only one or two topics at each clinic visit and to make a note of them in the patient's records.

Patients should be continually updated on new research and encouraged to join patient organizations, which also fulfil this role. Members of the diabetes team should be familiar and up-to-date with topics covered in patient magazines.

Monitoring glycaemic control

Glycaemic control is monitored in two ways:
- home monitoring by the patient
- laboratory monitoring.

All patients should be encouraged to undertake home monitoring and to record the results (see Chapter 4). A few (e.g. blind or demented patients) will be unable to carry out home monitoring, though a carer may be willing to help. If the patient is totally resistant to persuasion, more frequent laboratory monitoring (e.g. 3-monthly glycated haemoglobin measurements) may be the answer.

Home monitoring results should be reviewed and discussed with the patient. Time and effort are required to produce these records and lack of interest in them will rapidly demotivate the patient. Urine test results in patients with NIDDM should always be negative unless the patient has a low renal threshold. In general, for patients with IDDM, home blood glucose monitoring (HBGM) results should be 4–7 mmol/l before meals and less than 10 mmol/l after meals. Trends should be looked for and possible reasons considered.

Laboratory tests for glycaemic control include glycated haemoglobin (or fructosamine) determination (see page 13).

Discrepancies between HBGM results and laboratory tests may arise for several reasons:
- poor HBGM technique, which commonly leads to falsely low HBGM results due to too little blood on the test strip (see page 64)
- poor HBGM results and good laboratory test results, suggesting swinging blood glucose levels and possible asymptomatic hypoglycaemia

■ good HBGM results and poor laboratory results, suggesting either inaccurate or selective recording of blood glucose results – a common situation requiring tact and discretion.

The patient should be told the laboratory test results and given a full explanation of their implications. A record should be made in the patient's cooperation booklet (Figure 11.1; and see page 271) or shared care card (see page 33), and the patient may be congratulated, or given encouragement and support, as appropriate.

An individualized approach to attaining glycaemic targets

Recommended targets for glycaemic control are presented in Table 11.3. The good control category represents a gold standard that would be achieved in an ideal world. It should always be remembered, however, that:

■ there is no perfect treatment for diabetes

■ treatment may have significant side-effects (e.g. hypoglycaemia)

■ in certain patients, diabetes is difficult to control

■ diabetic patients have personal lives to cope with as well as diabetes

■ the patient's priorities and aspirations may differ from those of the health care professional.

Glycaemic targets need to be individualized to suit the patient, who will be motivated to improve further once a realistic target has been attained. Certain groups of patients warrant either very strict targets or more relaxed targets than the average patient.

■ Strict control is necessary in pregnant women (see Chapter 12).

■ The elderly and those with a short life expectancy may not have time to benefit from a reduced complication rate and may therefore merit more relaxed targets, though 'elderly' needs to be interpreted on an individual basis; a woman of 70 may have a life expectancy of 10 years.

■ Adolescent patients may find control difficult because of hormonal changes, which may be exacerbated by teenage dietary indiscretions.

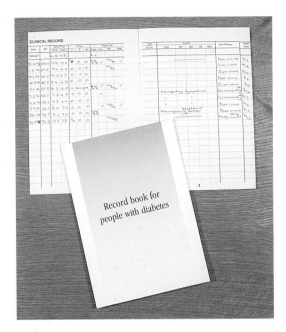

Figure 11.1 *Patient cooperation book.*

■ Good control may be dangerous in patients with hypoglycaemia unawareness, for whom safe control is paramount.

An inexplicable deterioration in glycaemic control requires investigation because it might be due to another illness (e.g. occult malignancy, recurrent urinary tract infection). Poor control may, of course, be due to a personal crisis for the patient, and this requires support and some temporary relaxation of glycaemic targets.

Monitoring weight

In the patient with NIDDM, weight control is a primary concern. Initial treatment may have been a weight-reducing diet. Subsequent weight gain is not uncommon and is likely to be accompanied by a deterioration in glycaemic control. The current targets for body mass index may be unattainable for some patients and may have to be modified in the light of a lifetime of being overweight.

Table 11.3 Targets for glycaemic control recommended by the British Diabetic Association[1]*

	Good	Acceptable	Poor	Very poor
HbA$_1$ (%); Normal 5.0–7.5	< 7.5	7.5–8.7	8.8–10.0	> 10.0
HbA$_{1C}$ (%); Normal 4.0–6.0	< 6.0	6.0–7.0	7.1–8.0	> 8.0
Fasting glucose (mmol/l)				
Plasma	< 7.0	7.1–7.8	7.9–9.0	> 9.0
Venous whole blood	< 6.0	6.0–7.0	7.1–8.0	> 8.0
Serum cholesterol (mmol/l)	< 5.2	5.2–6.4	6.5–7.8	> 7.8
Serum triglycerides (mmol/l)	< 1.7	1.7–2.2	2.3–4.4	> 4.4
Body mass index (kg/m²)	< 25	25.0–26.9	27.0–30.0	> 30
Systolic blood pressure (mm Hg)	< 140	140–159	160–180	> 180
Diastolic blood pressure (mm Hg)	< 90	91–94	95–100	> 100

*For targets suggested by European NIDDM Policy Group, see page 77.

NB: Each laboratory quotes its own normal range for HbA$_1$/HbA$_{1C}$. Targets have been calculated using mean + SD.

■ Good = < (mean + 2 SD)
■ Acceptable = < (mean + 4 SD)
■ Poor = < (mean + 6 SD)
■ Very poor > (mean + 6 SD)

To find out the mean and SD at your laboratory, either contact them directly or calculate indirectly. Most laboratories quote a normal range based on the mean ± 2 SD, so the mid-point of the normal range is the mean and the mid-point subtracted from the upper limit represents 2 SD.

In the insulin treated patient, weight gain in the face of poor control suggests poor dietary compliance. Control of body weight can be difficult for some insulin treated patients and strict dieting may be hazardous because of hypoglycaemia. Weight loss may be achieved by carefully reducing total calorie intake, spreading carbohydrate throughout the day and appropriate insulin dose reduction. This is best negotiated jointly between doctor, patient and dietitian.

Identification of risk factors for macrovascular disease

As diabetic patients are at increased risk of cardiovascular, cerebrovascular and peripheral vascular diseases (see Chapter 15), regular follow-up should include assessment of the risk factors for these diseases. Patients should be actively discouraged from smoking and the risks of smoking pointed out to them. Overemphasis on smoking must not, however, be allowed to upset the patient-doctor relationship.

Lipid levels should be regularly determined, and those patients who show hyperlipidaemia should be assessed on a 3–6-monthly basis.

The close correlation between the lipid profile and the degree of glycaemic control means that in a patient with deranged lipid levels, glycaemic control must be optimized first before considering drug treatment for hyperlipidaemia. Targets for lipid levels are presented on page 191 and in Table 11.3.

Hypertension is relatively common in patients with diabetes, particularly in older people with NIDDM who are likely to be over-weight. Blood pressure should be monitored routinely, with the patient sitting *and rested.* Thresholds for antihypertensive treatment in diabetic patients are below those for the population at large (see page 196 and Table 11.3).

Screening for complications

All patients should be screened annually for complications (retinopathy, nephropathy, neuropathy and diabetic foot disease; Table 11.1 and Chapters 13, 14, 16 and 17). The aim is to detect complications at an early and treatable stage and to refer to a specialist if appropriate.

Advice on treatment

Many forms of treatment may be commenced in primary care (e.g. oral hypoglycaemic agents, antihypertensive therapy, non-pharmaceutical options, such as exercise). The purpose of the treatment should always be fully explained to the patient, along with how drugs work and any possible side-effects.

Patients often find it difficult to remember all the information received during a consultation. Each patient should, therefore, have a record card or treatment book, which can be filled in with drug doses and notes to act as prompts.

Maintenance of patient morale

It is impossible to overemphasize the importance of maintaining patient morale. Although the initial grief reaction (see page 38) will probably be over by the time long-term care is under consideration, this is not always the case, and acceptance of the diabetes still may not have occurred. Even if it has, and coping strategies are in place, the patient may all too easily lose confidence, particularly in the light of poor glycaemic control. It is vital, therefore, that all diabetes team members work continually to encourage and support patients and help to maintain morale and self esteem. Treatment of the patient as an individual trying to cope with a lifelong disease rather than as just another case of diabetes is *so* important.

Arrangement of further follow-up

All diabetic patients require regular follow-up. Therefore, at the end of each visit, arrangements need to be made for the next consultation, with tests being completed beforehand so that results are available. Patients failing to attend should be contacted and a further appointment arranged.

Shared care summary

All diabetic patients require regular follow-up. Well-defined protocols should be followed for both routine clinic visits (Table 11.2) and for the annual review (Table 11.1), which may take place either in general practice or at hospital. The aims of follow-up are to:

■ encourage the patient's determination to undertake self care
■ teach and update the patient about all aspects of diabetes
■ monitor glycaemic control
■ monitor weight and general health
■ identify risk factors for macrovascular complications
■ screen regularly for all diabetic complications
■ advise on treatment
■ maintain patient morale and self esteem.

Reference

1 British Diabetic Association, Diabetes Services Advisory Committee. *Recommendations for the management of diabetes in primary care.* London: British Diabetic Association, 1993.

Further reading

Fox C, Pickering A. *Diabetes in the real world.* London: Class Publishing, 1995.

MacKinnon M. *Providing diabetes care in general practice. 2nd edn.* London: Class Publishing, 1995.

Chapter 12

Pregnancy, contraception and HRT

Over the last 50 years, the outlook for women with insulin dependent diabetes mellitus (IDDM) contemplating pregnancy has improved considerably. Perinatal mortality of babies of diabetic mothers has dropped significantly (Figure 12.1)[1], and the majority of pregnant diabetic women now give birth to healthy babies. A successful outcome is, however, achieved only through excellent glycaemic control preconception, careful control of diabetes during pregnancy and close obstetric supervision. Diabetic pregnancies are high-risk events in obstetric terms, and hospital supervision is essential for all pregnant

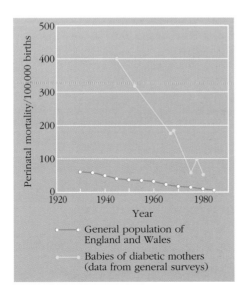

General population of
England and Wales

Babies of diabetic mothers
(data from general surveys)

Figure 12.1 *Decline in perinatal mortality among babies of diabetic mothers in England and Wales. Adapted from Lowy C, 1991*[1].

diabetic women. The primary health care team (PHCT) also needs to be involved, as during emergencies (e.g. severe hypoglycaemic attacks) the family practitioner will be called upon, and after the birth, the mother and baby need support. The patient herself must undertake the major role of monitoring her glycaemic control fastidiously.

In this chapter, guidelines are presented on the management of diabetes during pregnancy. The problem of gestational diabetes is discussed and a policy for screening is proposed. The chapter closes with a discussion of contraceptive methods and hormone replacement therapy (HRT) suitable for diabetic patients and the risks of children of diabetic parents becoming diabetic in turn.

Pregnancy and diabetes mellitus

The hormones produced by the placenta during pregnancy antagonize the effects of insulin. In non-diabetic women, endogenous insulin production is increased during pregnancy in order to compensate for these hormonal changes. Thus, problems of glycaemic control are common during pregnancy in diabetic women.

In the first trimester, swinging blood glucose levels are not unusual, with unpredictable hypoglycaemic episodes and rebound hyperglycaemia. During the second trimester, insulin requirements begin to rise, usually from about 18–20 weeks, climbing dramatically until about 32 weeks, when they often stabilize. Insulin requirements return to normal immediately after delivery and pregnancy has no long-term effect on the diabetes.

In a small number of diabetic women, pregnancy may be inadvisable because of the risk to the mother's health. Women with active proliferative retinopathy should delay pregnancy until laser photocoagulation has been completed. The advice of the ophthalmologist should be sought. Women with diabetic nephropathy are more likely to develop hypertension and obstetric complications. Those with significant impairment of renal function (serum creatinine > 200 µmol/l) should be advised against pregnancy, as it can be complicated by rapid deterioration in renal function necessitating renal dialysis.

The foetus and baby of a diabetic mother

The incidence of congenital abnormalities is higher among babies of diabetic mothers than among the general population. There is a correlation between the risk of abnormality and poor glycaemic control during the early weeks of pregnancy. This means that excellent glycaemic control prior to conception is important. Reassuringly, hypoglycaemia in the mother, even if severe, seldom seems to be a problem for the foetus. Good glycaemic control is not, however, the only factor involved. Even with good control, the risk of foetal abnormalities remains higher than in the non-diabetic population. A range of congenital abnormalities, similar to that arising in the general population, occurs in babies of diabetic mothers, though caudal regression syndrome is recognized as being specific to diabetes.

Spontaneous abortion is no more common among well controlled diabetic patients than among other mothers, but among poorly controlled patients, the abortion rate is higher, probably due to lethal developmental abnormalities (Figure 12.2)[2].

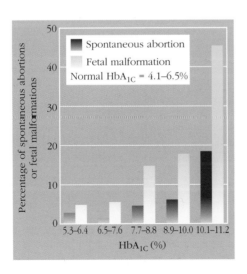

Figure 12.2 *Percentage cases of spontaneous abortion or fetal malformation in relation to glycated haemoglobin (HbA$_{1c}$) level at the 9th week of pregnancy in women with insulin dependent diabetes. Adapted from Hanson U et al., 1990[2].*

Later in pregnancy, problems of macrosomia, sudden intra-uterine death or occasionally intra-uterine growth retardation may arise. Macrosomia — a large fat baby with body weight above the 90th centile for gestational age (Figure 12.3) — is the most commonly encountered complication and is usually due to poor glycaemic control. High levels of glucose in the blood crossing the placenta prompt an increased insulin secretion in the foetus leading to increased growth and particularly fat deposition; such babies are at risk of sudden intra-uterine death.

During the first 48 hours after delivery, babies of diabetic mothers may develop hypoglycaemia due to excessive endogenous insulin secretion. This is particularly common when the maternal diabetes has not been well controlled. All babies of diabetic mothers are monitored closely, with 3-hourly blood glucose determinations for the first 48 hours.

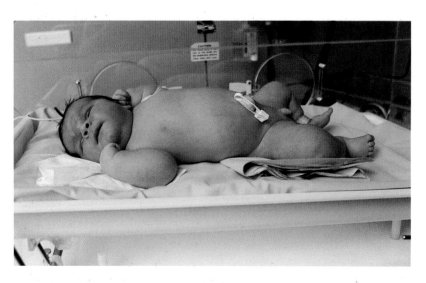

Figure 12.3 *Macrosomia: the most common complication of a pregnancy in which glycaemic control has been poor.*

Guidelines for managing diabetes in pregnancy

■ All diabetic women planning a pregnancy should be referred to the diabetologist for pre-pregnancy counselling to achieve excellent glycaemic control prior to conception. Those with non-insulin dependent diabetes mellitus (NIDDM) treated with oral hypoglycaemic agents need to be changed to insulin as soon as pregnancy is contemplated. Standard preconception counselling (e.g. concerning rubella protection and adequate folate intake) also needs to be given.

■ All diabetic women with a confirmed pregnancy should be referred for hospital assessment and supervision, preferably to a unit with a joint obstetric clinic. Follow-up will be at least every 2 weeks for the duration of the pregnancy.

■ Excellent glycaemic control should be the aim, with HbA_{1c} in the normal range, preprandial blood glucose in the range 4–6 mmol/l and 2-hours postprandial blood glucose below 9 mmol/l.

■ Home blood glucose monitoring should be undertaken four times a day every day for the duration of the pregnancy.

■ A full dietary reappraisal is essential to ensure regular carbohydrate intake for the avoidance of hypoglycaemia and to fulfil the nutritional demands of pregnancy.

■ The patient and her partner should be educated about avoiding and treating hypoglycaemia, and glucagon should be prescribed, if appropriate.

■ An early ultrasound scan should be undertaken for confirmation of gestation age; another scan is carried out at 18–20 weeks to check for foetal abnormality. From 28–36 weeks, scans are undertaken every 2 weeks to monitor foetal growth.

■ Breast feeding should be encouraged but usually requires a 10% reduction in insulin dose plus additional carbohydrate snacks.

Gestational diabetes

The hormonal changes in pregnancy lead to increasing insulin production by the pancreas of the pregnant woman. In some women, the pancreas is unable to cope with the additional demands, blood glucose levels rise and diabetes develops. Occasionally, 'true' diabetic patients present in pregnancy. Although this may be suspected, it can be confirmed only by a postpartum glucose tolerance test. Gestational diabetes resolves following delivery, but these patients have a significant risk of developing diabetes in the future.

There remains considerable debate about the need to screen for diabetes in pregnancy[3]. The enthusiasts believe that it is important to detect and intervene in all such cases of glucose intolerance and diabetes. The doubters rightly claim that there is no evidence of reduction in perinatal morbidity or mortality when screening is instituted. Screening detects many women with only minor glucose intolerance and may cause undue anxiety for such women. The preferred strategy is to screen high-risk women and maintain a high index of suspicion in the remainder. A more formal screening programme may be appropriate in areas with greater proportions of ethnic monorities; Asian and Aboriginal women, for example, have a higher incidence of gestational diabetes than Caucasian women.

Suggested policy for gestational diabetes screening

A glucose tolerance test (GTT) should be organized for 28 weeks for patients at high risk of gestational diabetes, namely those with:

- a history of gestational diabetes in a previous pregnancy (see below)
- a previous baby weighing over 4 kg at birth
- a family history of diabetes mellitus (in a first degree relative)
- obesity (body mass index over 28 kg/m^2 at booking)
- a previous unexplained stillbirth.

Pregnancy may cause a lowering of the renal glucose threshold, so glycosuria is not uncommonly detected in the routine urine tests. Diabetes should always be excluded. Women with a previous history of gestational diabetes should have a laboratory random plasma glucose measurement at the booking visit and at approximately 18–20 weeks. If the plasma glucose is above 6 mmol/l, a GTT should immediately be arranged. Otherwise, it should be undertaken at 28 weeks.

It is worth noting that due to the changing hormone levels during pregnancy, a normal result early in pregnancy does not preclude the subsequent development of gestational diabetes.

Management plan for IGT and gestational diabetes

During pregnancy

■ Refer all patients to the dietitian for assessment and advice.

■ Refer to the joint obstetric clinic (or diabetologist and obstetrician).

■ Excellent glycaemic control should be achieved with similar guidelines for established diabetic patients. Those failing to achieve this with diet alone need to commence insulin treatment.

After delivery

■ Discontinue all insulin treatment and continue to monitor blood glucose levels for 24–48 hours.

■ Organize a GTT, either while the patient is still on the postnatal ward or at 6 weeks after delivery.

■ Advise about beneficial lifestyle changes to regain ideal body weight and maintain exercise.

■ Advise on the risk of diabetes development during future pregnancies.

■ Advise on risk of developing diabetes in future and recommend annual 2-hour postprandial laboratory blood glucose determination for early detection of diabetes.

Interpretation of GTT in pregnancy

The interpretation of the GTT should follow that outlined for the diagnosis of diabetes (see page 23). Some experts do not apply the term impaired glucose tolerance (IGT) to pregnant women, but classify all pregnant women with IGT as having gestational diabetes.

Contraception and HRT in women with diabetes

Recognizing the problems associated with diabetes in pregnancy and particularly the increased congenital abnormality rate, it is important that all pregnancies should be planned. As fertility is not impaired by diabetes, early and appropriate contraceptive advice is imperative for teenagers and women with diabetes.

Physical barrier methods, such as condoms or caps, are suitable. Their success depends on a high level of motivation in the couple. Intra-uterine coil devices may also be used as their efficacy is no longer believed to be lower in diabetic women. They should be avoided, however, in the presence of pelvic infection.

Many patients prefer an oral contraceptive preparation, in which case the progesterone-only pill is the best choice for diabetic women. The combined oral contraceptive pill containing synthetic oestrogens carries an increased risk of arterial disease. As diabetic patients already have an increased risk of vascular disease, the combined pill should be avoided if possible, and particularly in patients who smoke, who are aged over 35 years, who have diabetic complications (e.g. retinopathy or nephropathy), who are overweight or have a family history of macrovascular disease.

The choice of contraceptive must be made jointly with the patient and preferably with her partner. Avoidance of an unplanned pregnancy may be the overriding concern in certain cases (e.g. teenagers). The failure rate of the progesterone-only pill, although low, or its narrow margin for error may preclude its use. If the combined oral contraceptive pill is then the method of choice, a pill with as low a dose of oestrogen as possible (20–30 μg/day) is preferable. When commencing treatment, a small increase in insulin dose (2–4 units/day) may be required. Patients should be warned to monitor blood glucose more closely during the first few weeks and adjust the insulin dose appropriately. In an established couple, a small risk of pregnancy may be acceptable and the progesterone-only pill or a barrier method may be suitable.

It is important to review the choice of contraceptive with the patient at regular intervals. In view of the risks of arterial disease associated with synthetic oestrogens, it would be advisable to try to limit the duration of use of the combined pill to less than 10 years. For an established couple not wanting children, a diabetic woman may be offered sterilization, or her partner a vasectomy.

Diabetes mellitus is no contraindication to the use of HRT. In fact, HRT has a beneficial effect with respect to the possible development of ischaemic heart disease and stroke, to which diabetic women are at increased risk. For patients with an intact uterus, the progestogen component of the HRT should be chosen with minimal lipid disturbance in mind (see page 192).

Risk of diabetes in the offspring

Many diabetic women worry about the risk of their children developing diabetes. In general, this risk is small, and diabetes is never present at birth. One study reported a cumulative risk of diabetes development of 6.3% by the age of 34 years if one parent has IDDM[4]. Recent evidence suggests that the risk may be higher if the father, rather than the mother, has IDDM (6.1% vs 1.3%)[5].

Shared care summary

■ Although pregnancy planning is essential for diabetic mothers, with adequate care and supervision, there is a good chance of a healthy baby. Both the PHCT and the hospital diabetes team should be closely involved in the care of a pregnant woman with diabetes.

■ All diabetic women of childbearing age should be made aware of the importance of planned pregnancies and should receive advice on contraception.

■ All diabetic women considering a pregnancy should be referred to the diabetologist and the hospital team. Pre-pregnancy counselling to achieve excellent glycaemic control is essential.

■ Pregnancy should be confirmed by the family practitioner, who should refer the patient at an early stage to the antenatal clinic and the diabetologist – preferably to a joint diabetic obstetric clinic.

■ The PHCT may be called on to deal with episodes of severe hypoglycaemia during pregnancy.

■ Diabetic women should be asked to monitor blood glucose closely (four tests/day) throughout pregnancy with the aim of achieving excellent control (HbA_{1C} within the normal range).

■ Attendance at a hospital clinic at least every 2 weeks throughout pregnancy is advisable.

■ Gestational diabetes may be diagnosed in primary care when there is a high index of suspicion. Referral to the diabetologist and dietitian is appropriate. Gestational diabetes resolves following pregnancy, but such women are at increased risk of future development of diabetes, so an annual laboratory 2-hour postprandial plasma glucose should be undertaken.

References

1 Lowy C. Pregnancy. In: Pickup EJ, Williams G, eds. *Textbook of diabetes*. Oxford: Blackwell Scientific Publications, 1991: 835–50.

2 Hanson U, Persson B, Thunell S. Relationship between haemoglobin A_{1c} in early Type 1 (insulin-dependent) diabetic pregnancy and the occurrence of spontaneous abortion and fetal malformation in Sweden. *Diabetologia* 1990; **33:** 100–4.

3 Ales KL, Santini DL. Should all pregnant women be screened for gestational glucose intolerance? *Lancet* 1989; **i:** 1187–91.

4 Lorenzen T, Pociot F, Hougaard P, Nerup J. Long-term risk of IDDM in first degree relatives of patients with IDDM. *Diabetologia* 1994; **37:** 321–7.

5 Warnam JN, Krowleski AS, Gottlieb MS *et al.* Differences in risk of insulin-dependent diabetes in offspring of diabetic mothers and fathers. *N Engl J Med* 1984; **311:** 149–52.

Further reading

Knopfler A. *Diabetes and pregnancy*. London: MacDonald Optima, 1989.

Chapter 13

Diabetic eye disease

The importance of eye disease in diabetes lies in the simple fact that diabetes is the single most common cause of blindness in the 20–60-year age group. This chapter briefly summarizes the ocular manifestations of diabetes, the size of the problem, its detection and treatment. In no other aspect of diabetes care is integrated shared care more important.

Ocular manifestations of diabetes mellitus

The ocular manifestations of diabetes are summarized in Table 13.1. The transient refractory changes are related to swings in blood glucose concentration and can lead to reduced visual acuity during episodes of very poor control. This condition is not uncommon at diagnosis and may be a presenting symptom. Astute optometrists often diagnose diabetes on the basis of rapid changes in visual acuity occurring over a period of days. It is sensible for spectacles not to be dispensed until glycaemic control is stable.

Young patients with insulin dependent diabetes (IDDM) may develop lens opacities (Figure 13.1), which are clearly visible on examination, though their presence is uncommon. As these opacities are polar in position – so-called juvenile cataract – visual acuity is severely affected. These lens opacities usually occur after a period of severe metabolic disturbance with hyperglycaemia. The high intracellular osmolarity (probably related to sorbitol retention) produces marked disruption of the lens structure and severe

Table 13.1 Ocular manifestations of diabetes mellitus

Early manifestations
- Transient refractory changes related to osmolarity
- Diabetic cataract

Late manifestations
- Accelerated senile cataract
- Diabetic retinopathy and its complications
- Ocular motor palsies resulting from mononeuritis (see Chapter 16)

Complications of diabetic retinopathy
- Maculopathy
- Vitreous haemorrhage/membrane formation
- Traction retinal detachment
- Rubeotic glaucoma

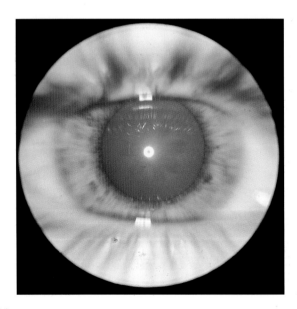

Figure 13.1 *Polar cataract in a juvenile patient with IDDM.*

refractory error. With good glycaemic control, such cataracts may disappear spontaneously allowing the restoration of visual acuity. If permanent damage to the lens has occurred, cataract extraction may be necessary.

Accelerated senile cataract (Figure 13.2) is very common, in contrast to the occurrence of juvenile cataract. Senile cataracts are usually initially situated in the periphery of the lens and have the appearance of roman numerals on a clock face. Visual acuity is spared initially, but with time, the opacities expand until they encroach on the optical axis of the lens causing a diminution in visual acuity. Small opacities at the posterior pole of the lens can produce severe loss of visual acuity. Diabetic patients with significant lens opacities should be referred for cataract extraction. Otherwise, screening for diabetic retinopathy may be adversely affected.

Diabetic retinopathy and its complications

At any one time, about 26–35% of diabetic patients have retinopathy (Table 13.2).

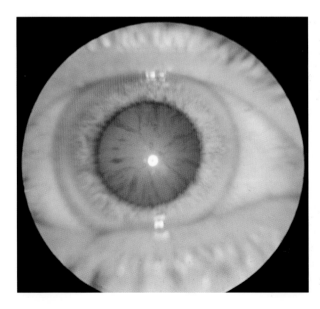

Figure 13.2 *Senile cataract common in older diabetic patients; does not differ from cataracts seen in non-diabetic elderly patients.*

Table 13.2 Prevalence of diabetic eye disease*

	Diabetes	Any retinopathy	Serious retinopathy**	Blindness
Percentage	1.5	26–35	9.5–11.0	1–2
†Number/250,000 people	3750	975–1312	356–412	37–75
‡Number/2000 people	30	8–24	3	0 or 1

*Gatling W, Hill RD; unpublished data.
**Retinopathy is defined as serious if it is sight threatening and requires treatment.
†Average hospital district.
‡Possible family practitioner list size.

Factors affecting the development and evolution of retinopathy

Family practitioners and hospital doctors caring for patients with diabetes need to be aware of the risk factors for retinopathy, which include:

- long duration of diabetes
- uncontrolled hypertension
- chronic renal failure
- poor glycaemic control.

Uncontrolled hypertension, particularly raised systolic blood pressure, adversely affects retinopathy, often accelerating its progression. Chronic renal failure is also associated with rapidly deteriorating retinopathy, probably due to fluid retention and hypertension. Good glycaemic control may prevent or retard the development of retinopathy in the early stages. This has been clearly shown for IDDM in the Diabetes Control and Complications Trial (DCCT)[1]. The transition from poor glycaemic control to excellent glycaemic control may, however, lead to a transient worsening of retinopathy.

Definitions of retinal appearances

Characteristic changes associated with diabetic retinopathy are shown in Figures 13.3–13.8. Although retinal appearances have been described in many ways, the definitions given in Table 13.3 have proved useful in practice. Particular attention should be paid to the shape, sharpness of outline, colour, size and other associated features of the components of retinopathy.

Diagnosis of retinopathy is not always straightforward even when the condition is serious. For example, diabetic maculopathy, which causes a decrease in central visual acuity that is not corrected by refraction or a pinhole, is difficult to diagnose though it demands prompt referral to an ophthalmologist.

Classification of diabetic retinopathy based on retinal appearance

The diverse appearances of diabetic retinopathy may be broadly classified into four groups (Table 13.4). This subdivision helps to clarify the significance, prognosis, need for follow-up and indications for treatment.

All diabetic patients are at risk of developing diabetic retinopathy, though the degree of development depends to some extent on the duration of diabetes. The time of onset of diabetes may be difficult to determine for non-insulin dependent diabetes (NIDDM), in which hyperglycaemia may have been present for months or even years before diagnosis (see page 245). Some 10% of such patients already have background retinopathy (Figure 13.3) at the time of diagnosis. Indeed, some patients may present with exudative maculopathy (Figure 13.4) as their first symptomatic feature of diabetes. Retinopathy is seldom present at diagnosis of IDDM, though blinding retinopathy at presentation has been recorded. Background retinopathy is the anticipated finding after 15–20 years of IDDM.

The risk of progression from good vision to blindness depends to some extent on the age at onset of the diabetes and the type of retinopathy.

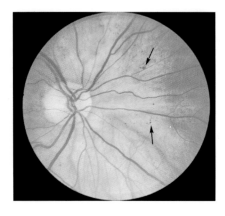

Figure 13.3 *Minimal background retinopathy with dots and blots (arrows) only.*

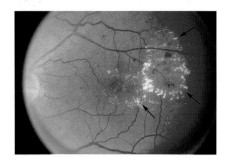

Figure 13.4 *Exudative maculopathy. Circinate exudate rings (arrows) from leaking microaneurysms. Dots, blots and haemorrhage also present. Refer for laser treatment.*

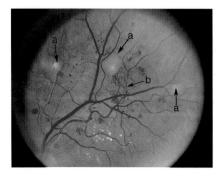

Figure 13.5 *Preproliferative retinopathy. Cotton wool spots (retinal infarcts; arrows a) and intraretinal microvascular abnormalities (IRMA; arrow b). Dots, blots, haemorrhages and exudates also present. Refer to ophthalmologist for close supervision.*

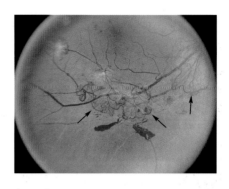

Figure 13.6 *Proliferative retinopathy. New vessels (arrows) in the peripheral retina. Haemorrhage and cotton wool spots also present. Refer to ophthalmologist for laser treatment.*

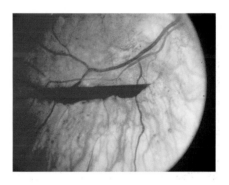

Figure 13.7 *Sub-hyaloid haemorrhage indicates bleeding from proliferative retinopathy. New vessels not visible here. Urgent referral to ophthalmologist required.*

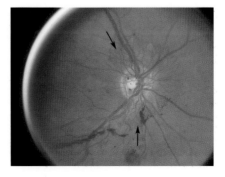

Figure 13.8 *Proliferative retinopathy. New vessels at the optic disc (arrows). Dots and blots also present but note paucity of other features of retinopathy. Proliferative retinopathy can appear with relatively few other visible features. Requires urgent referral to ophthalmologist for laser treatment.*

Table 13.3 Definitions of the components of diabetic retinopathy

Feature	Type	Appearance
Dots	Microaneurysms or microhaemorrhages	Small, round, red lesions
Blots	Haemorrhages	Medium sized (<1500 µm), round, red lesions with an indistinct outline
Hard exudates	Oedema/lipid deposits	Irregular, yellowish-white deposits with sharp outline.* Often in circinate patterns
Cotton wool spots	Ischaemic areas	White or grey areas with indistinct outlines, which may be surrounded by haemorrhage, dilated capillaries or large microaneurysms**
New vessels	New vessels	Usually a fine tangled mass of vessels indicating that retinopathy has progressed to the proliferative stage, which is sight threatening

*Must be distinguished from colloid bodies (drusen), which are small, round yellowish berry-like lesions not related to diabetes.
**Often associated with other signs of ischaemia, including intraretinal microvascular abnormalities (IRMA), venous dilatation, venous beading and looping.

Other vascular abnormalities	■ Venous changes	■ Gross venous dilatation with irregularity, beading and looping, suggesting severe ischaemia
	■ Capillary closure	■ Areas of dull, atrophic retina
	■ Arterial changes	■ Irregular vessel diameters and wall sheathing
Haemorrhages (other than dots or blots)		Red lesions: ■ flame shaped ■ boat shaped ■ diffuse[†] ■ vitreous, lying within the vitreous, obscuring the retina[‡] ■ deep, dark, round haemorrhages with a clear, sharp outline
Maculopathy	■ Ischaemic changes in the macula	■ Atrophic macula Difficult to detect
	■ Oedematous changes in the macula[§]	■ Swollen macula area Difficult to detect

[†]Indicating severe ischaemia.
[‡]Indicating bleeding from new vessels.
[§]Suspicions of macula oedema are raised by hard exudates within the temporal triangle.

Table 13.4 Classification of diabetic retinopathy on ophthalmoscopy

Class of retinopathy	Features
Background retinopathy	Dots, blots, hard exudates, haemorrhages, up to 5 cotton wool spots
Preproliferative retinopathy	Dots and blots, > 5 cotton wool spots, with or without areas of capillary closure (± hard exudates), deep dark round haemorrhages, sheet haemorrhages, IRMA, venous abnormalities
Proliferative retinopathy	Peripheral new vessels, disc new vessels, with or without fibrous proliferation (retinitis proliferans)
Maculopathy	Ischaemia or oedema of the macular area

IRMA = intraretinal microvascular abnormalities.

Multiple (more than five) cotton wool spots (Figure 13.5) are highly suggestive of new vessel development within 2 years and this is why a severely ischaemic retina is classified as preproliferative.

The risk of developing severe visual impairment in the 2 years following the discovery of peripheral new vessels (Figure 13.6) ranges from 7 to 30%. The degree of risk depends on the extent of new vessel formation and the presence of vitreous or preretinal haemorrhage. The risk of developing severe visual impairment during the 2 years following the discovery of disc new vessels is as great as 10–40%. Again, this depends on the presence and extent of vitreous or preretinal haemorrhage.

The 5-year incidence of blindness in patients with untreated proliferative retinopathy is a dramatic 60%. Proliferative retinopathy carries with it the danger of vitreous haemorrhage; 30% of patients with untreated proliferative retinopathy who have a vitreous haemorrhage are blind within a year.

If blindness is to be prevented, the following actions are necessary:
- early diagnosis of diabetes
- early detection of background retinopathy
- regular follow-up of patients with retinopathy in order to detect any significant progression
- early referral for assessment and treatment before significant loss of visual acuity
- prompt and appropriate laser photocoagulation of sight threatening retinopathy.

Screening for diabetic eye disease: whose responsibility?

The coordination, integration and organization of the screening service may be the responsibility of either a diabetologist or an ophthalmologist. Any screening programme must reach the majority of the diabetic population. Good compliance is essential, so the service must be convenient for patients and must have both an annual recall system and a built-in protocol for dealing with non-attenders. The person responsible for the district service must, therefore, ensure the efficient development and operation of a district diabetes register and a central reporting system. The communication system between primary and secondary care must be foolproof. Criteria for recall of patients screening positive must be clearly defined, as should the pathway for further follow-up and treatment.

If an efficient screening programme does not exist in the area, family practitioners should press for its institution or attempt to screen for retinopathy in general practice (see panel), a procedure that is not without pitfalls. Litigation for missed retinopathy may prove expensive. Therefore, the practitioner needs to consider carefully whether he/she is competent for the job; good postgraduate eye

Essential features of screening for diabetic retinopathy

■ Operate an annual recall system.

■ Measure distant visual acuity with Snellen chart (or similar). Use spectacles or pinhole to correct refractive errors.

■ Dilate pupils with a mydriatic agent (1% tropicamide). Ensure dilatation is adequate for good retinal views. Maculopathy cannot be excluded without adequate pupil dilatation.

■ In a darkened room, examine both retinae, including the macular area, either by direct ophthalmoscopy or by retinal photography.

■ Document the results of the examination and inform the patient and the health care professional supervising diabetes care.

■ Refer to an ophthalmologist for further assessment those patients found to have:

– sight threatening retinopathy (see text)

– significant progression of retinopathy (see text)

– an inadequate screening examination (e.g. due to lens opacity).

■ Prompt non-attenders and inform health care professionals supervising diabetes care. Audit results of screening.

training is advisable. An alternative is to contact the local optometrist and ensure that the eye examination is correctly executed (see panel).

Prevention and treatment of diabetic retinopathy

Prevention

Most diabetologists now believe that hyperglycaemia plays a major role in the causation of diabetic retinopathy. Various studies have shown a correlation between the prevalence of retinopathy and poor glycaemic control. Detection of diabetes in its early stages, regular follow-up and the maintenance of good glycaemic control must, therefore, be the primary aims for retinopathy prevention. General measures, such as good blood pressure control, anti-smoking education and the normalization of blood lipids should also be undertaken. Screening for diabetic eye disease should be carried out annually without fail and should follow the recall policy outlined in Table 13.5. Local policy may dictate the appropriate referral route to ensure prompt assessment. However, it is advisable that patients who are recalled for further investigation should be seen by a diabetologist experienced in eye examination, thus protecting the ophthalmologist from unnecessary referrals. This procedure also provides the opportunity for a full review of the patient's diabetes. Retinopathy is a marker for other complications; the patient should not be treated merely as a pair of eyes.

In one primary screening programme for diabetic eye disease[2], 6% of the screened patients were recalled. About 25% of these patients were referred for ophthalmological opinion in the Joint Diabetic Eye Clinic, and nearly half required laser therapy.

Treatment by photocoagulation

Laser photocoagulation has traditionally been carried out in the outpatient clinic of the ophthalmology department, but the advent of portable lasers allows it to be undertaken in diabetes centres. Patients need reassurance that the treatment is neither difficult nor painful. The laser beam appears merely as a bright flash to the patient seated at a slit lamp.

For maculopathy, photocoagulation usually consists of the application of a small number of laser burns to the leaking capillaries causing the exudates and oedema. The treatment is relatively quick, taking only about 5–10 minutes for 50–200 burns/eye.

For proliferative retinopathy, photocoagulation needs to be far more extensive as laser burns need to be applied to a large part of the peripheral retina (i.e. pan-photocoagulation) to destroy the ischaemic

Table 13.5 Advisable recall policy for diabetic eye screening

Feature	Recall policy
Dots and blots only	No recall
Exudates	Recall if new feature
Exudates in temporal triangle	Recall
Haemorrhage	Recall if new feature
Cotton wool spots	Recall
Proliferative retinopathy	Urgent recall
Vitreous haemorrhage	Urgent recall
Maculopathy	Urgent recall

areas (Figure 13.9). Several laser sessions may be needed, as each eye may receive 3000–5000 burns. Some patients find this increasingly uncomfortable at each session, and for these, a retrobulbar local anaesthetic may be given. Successful laser treatment leads to a shrivelling and disappearance of the new vessels over a few weeks.

Close observation by the ophthalmologist is necessary after laser therapy to confirm improvement in the condition of the retina.

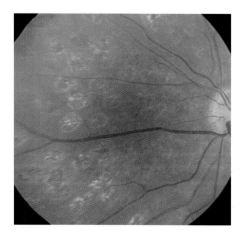

Figure 13.9 *Photocoagulation scars in a patient after successful treatment by pan-retinal ablation for proliferative retinopathy.*

Occasionally, particularly with maculopathy, further laser treatment is required. Laser therapy seldom leads to improved visual acuity. It may help to maintain reasonable vision, preventing blindness in 60% of sight threatened patients provided that the retinopathy is detected early while visual acuity is still good. Most patients treated by pan-photocoagulation are aware of reduced night vision and are dazzled by bright sunlight. Some may have a significant field loss, which may affect driving. Others notice a distinct reduction in the overall quality of vision despite the absence of deterioration in visual acuity.

Shared care summary

■ Diabetic eye disease is a common cause of blindness, though loss of vision is now largely preventable by laser photocoagulation therapy.

■ Transient changes in visual acuity due to swinging blood glucose levels are not uncommon at diagnosis or times of poor glycaemic control.

■ All new patients require an eye examination as diabetic retinopathy may be present even at diagnosis in patients with NIDDM.

■ An annual screening examination to detect retinopathy is essential.

■ Early detection of retinopathy is vital, as laser treatment is most successful if given before visual acuity is significantly reduced (i.e. when retinopathy is still asymptomatic).

■ Good glycaemic control may prevent the development of diabetic eye disease.

■ Regular monitoring of blood pressure and aggressive treatment of hypertension, best undertaken in primary care, is important in patients with diabetic retinopathy.

References

1 The Diabetes Control and Complications Trial Research Group. The effect of intensive treatment of diabetes on the development and progression of long-term complications in insulin-dependent diabetes mellitus. *N Engl J Med* 1993; **329:** 977–86.

2 Gatling W, Howie AJ, Hill RD. An optical practice based diabetic eye screening programme. *Diabet Med* 1995; **12:** 532–6.

Further reading

Ariffin A, Hill RD, Leigh O, eds. *Diabetes and primary eye care.* Oxford: Blackwell Scientific Books, 1992.

Kohner EM, Porta M, eds. *Screening for diabetic retinopathy in Europe: a field guidebook.* Copenhagen: WHO, Regional Office for Europe, 1992.

Chapter 14

Diabetic renal disease

Nephropathy is a common complication of diabetes and, if untreated, leads to end stage renal disease and death. The characteristic feature of nephropathy is the presence of protein in the urine. Symptoms are evident only late in this complication when there is renal failure.

This chapter considers the earliest stage of diabetic renal disease, microalbuminuria, and discusses the detection, assessment and treatment of patients with this condition in order to delay the progression to frank proteinuria. The clinical features of nephropathy are outlined, and the assessment and management of patients discussed. Although certain aspects demand referral to hospital specialists, screening and diagnosis are carried out in primary care, but treatment, particularly blood pressure control, is best undertaken through shared care.

Microalbuminuria

Definition
Microalbuminuria is defined as an albumin excretion rate (AER) above normal but below that detectable by certain dip-stick methods (e.g. Albustix®). In a timed overnight urine collection, microalbuminuria is an AER of 20–200 μg/minute. Diabetic patients with an AER above 200 μg/minute generally have established renal disease and frank proteinuria detectable by a dip-stick, such as Albustix®.

Microalbuminuria is not diagnostic of diabetic nephropathy; other renal diseases, such as glomerulonephritis, lead to a raised AER. It is also found in patients with hypertension, even if not diabetic, and in those with cardiovascular disease.

Significance of microalbuminuria

In patients with insulin dependent diabetes mellitus (IDDM), microalbuminuria has been shown to predict the development of future diabetic nephropathy, while in non-insulin dependent diabetes mellitus (NIDDM), it predicts not only nephropathy but also premature death from cardiovascular or cerebrovascular disease. This is probably due to the development of hypertension and its sequelae in older patients.

Microalbuminuria usually represents the earliest evidence of renal damage. Pathological changes in the glomeruli are visible on renal biopsy. However, microalbuminuria has also been found to occur temporarily in patients with uncontrolled diabetes (e.g. during intercurrent infection or at initial diagnosis). In such patients, improvement in glycaemic control often leads to normalization of AER. This may be due to reversible alteration in the glomerular filtration barrier due to change in charge, transport mechanisms or intracapillary pressure.

Screening for microalbuminuria

The benefits of screening for and treating microalbuminuria take 5–10 years to accrue. It is not acceptable, therefore, to screen patients who will not benefit during their lifetime. Screening tests in elderly patients are subject to error due to urinary tract infection (UTI), prostatic disease and heart failure, all of which may cause raised AER unrelated to diabetic nephropathy.

Urinary albumin excretion is known to vary in health and disease, with day-to-day variation up to 40%. Daytime AER is approximately 25% higher than night-time; exercise also increases AER in diabetic patients. Taking all of these factors into account, screening for microalbuminuria (Figure 14.1) is best carried out on an early morning urine sample[1] (i.e. the first specimen the patient passes on rising from bed).

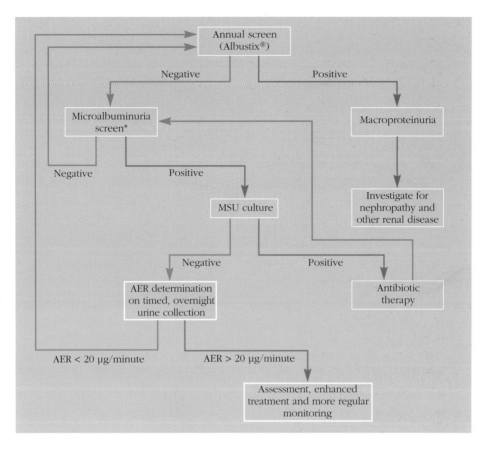

Figure 14.1 *A screening programme for microalbuminuria in patients with diabetes.*
MSU = mid-stream urine; AER = albumin excretion rate.
An early morning urine, excluding patients over 70 years of age, patients with short life expectancy, patients with decompensated diabetes and pregnant women.

Screening tests can be done in primary care using dip-stick methods, such as Micral-Test® or Bumintest®, or sent to the local laboratory. A positive microalbuminuria screen is usually based on an albumin concentration of at least 20 mg/l or an albumin:creatinine ratio greater than 2 mg/mol. Table 14.1 shows the prevalence of microalbuminuria in diabetic patients.

Table 14.1 Prevalence of microalbuminuria (i.e. albumin excretion rate at least 20 µg/minute) among diabetic patients

Type of patient	Prevalence (%)
IDDM	10
NIDDM	14
IDDM of 15 years' duration (diagnosed in childhood)	24

Assessment of the patient with microalbuminuria

Once microalbuminuria has been confirmed and a UTI excluded (Figure 14.1), referral to the specialist diabetologist is appropriate. A full assessment of the patient should include screening for other complications, because microalbuminuria has been shown to predict proliferative retinopathy and is commonly associated with a poor lipid profile. A full assessment should consist of:

- a full history of previous renal disease (e.g. renal calculi, glomerulonephritis, UTI)
- a history of macrovascular disease and hypertension
- a history of cigarette smoking and alcohol intake
- appraisal of diabetes management
- a full examination, including
  - blood pressure
  - cardiovascular, peripheral vascular and cerebrovascular systems
  - eyes (pupil dilatation and fundoscopy for retinopathy)
  - feet, for neuropathy and diabetic foot disease
- investigations, including
  - glucose, glycated haemoglobin, serum creatinine, lipid profile
  - ECG
  - renal tract ultrasound.

With such variability in AER, it is wise to organize two or three timed overnight urine collections to obtain a valid assessment of baseline microalbuminuria. Thereafter, AER should be measured every 3 months to monitor progress.

The aims of patient management are to:

■ optimize glycaemic control
■ treat hypertension aggressively with therapy that includes an angiotensin converting enzyme (ACE) inhibitor
■ reduce AER by using an ACE inhibitor in normotensive patients
■ reduce macrovascular disease risks by treating hyperlipidaemia, reducing smoking, etc.

Lowering blood pressure by any means will lead to a reduction in AER, but ACE inhibitors appear to have specific benefit in microalbuminuria and should be included in the antihypertensive regimen (see page 174) unless contraindicated (see page 198). Normotensive patients show a reduction in AER when treated with an ACE inhibitor (e.g. enalapril, 20 mg/day; Figure 14.2), without any change in blood pressure[2]. A recent study over 4 years in normotensive patients with NIDDM and microalbuminuria compared enalapril, 5 mg/day, with placebo. There was a significant reduction in AER in the actively treated group, whereas there was progression of the albuminuria with placebo[3].

Diabetic nephropathy

Definition
Diabetic nephropathy is defined clinically by the presence of persistent proteinuria (at least 500 mg/24 hours) in a diabetic patient with features of retinopathy but with no evidence of other renal tract disease.

Clinical features and natural history of diabetic renal disease
The earliest sign of renal damage is detected as microalbuminuria, which later progresses to overt proteinuria. Only a few patients develop severe proteinuria (at least 5 g/24 hours) sufficient to cause

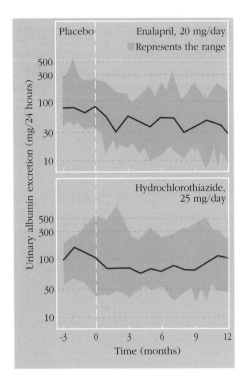

Figure 14.2 *Urinary albumin excretion falls in normotensive diabetic patients on treatment with the ACE inhibitor, enalapril, but not with hydrochlorothiazide (p < 0.05). Reproduced with permission from Hallab M et al., 1993[2].*

the nephrotic syndrome (i.e. the triad of proteinuria, hypoalbuminaemia and oedema, which is commonly associated with hypercholesterolaemia). These patients usually follow a rapidly progressive course and are highly symptomatic.

Once the stage of persistent proteinuria has been reached, the renal damage progresses and results in a fall in glomerular filtration rate (GFR). The rate of decline in GFR appears to be constant for any individual, but there is wide variation between patients (Figure 14.3)[4]. Hypertension is one of the most important factors determining the decline in GFR. Aggressive treatment can retard the process considerably (Figure 14.4)[5] and ACE inhibitors seem to be particularly effective (Figure 14.5)[6].

Patients with nephropathy invariably have accompanying retinopathy. As retinopathy can progress rapidly in a patient with

Diabetic nephropathy and IDDM*

■ Seldom occurs during the first 5 years of IDDM.

■ The annual incidence peaks at 3% after 15–17 years of diabetes. After 40 years' diabetes, the annual incidence is less than 1%.

■ Commoner in men than women, with a male:female ratio of 1.7:1. After more than 40 years' diabetes, 46% of men have nephropathy, compared with 32% of women.

■ The age at diagnosis influences the risk: highest risk in those diagnosed from 11–20 years, of whom 44% develop nephropathy.

■ Following the onset of persistent proteinuria, 25% develop end-stage renal failure after 6 years and 75% after 15 years.

■ After 40 years' diabetes, only 10% of patients developing proteinuria are alive, compared with 70% of those without proteinuria.

■ Before 1942, 41% of patients developed nephropathy after 25–30 years of diabetes; since 1949 the figure has dropped to 25%.

*See Further reading for details.

Diabetic nephropathy and NIDDM

■ Proteinuria may be present at diagnosis.

■ The prevalence of proteinuria increases with duration of NIDDM: 7–10% during the first 5 years and 20–35% between 20 and 25 years' NIDDM.

■ A history of hypertension before onset of proteinuria is not uncommon.

■ A history of parental diabetic nephropathy is predictive of nephropathy.

■ Many patients die from heart disease or stroke before reaching end stage renal failure.

nephropathy, fundoscopy should be undertaken at least every 6 months. Progression in a matter of months from simple background retinopathy to proliferative retinopathy is not unusual.

Patients with diabetes generally show poor tolerance of uraemia and end stage renal failure. Fluid retention and heart failure are problematic from an early stage, often before the serum creatinine has reached 500 μmol/l. Renal support, in the form of dialysis or transplantation, needs to be considered before there is significant deterioration in general health. Other relatively common problems are significant neuropathy and peripheral vascular disease leading to diabetic foot disease. By this stage, the body is scarcely able to resist infection, and sepsis commonly leads to amputation. Many older diabetic patients succumb to heart disease or stroke before reaching advanced renal failure.

Screening for and diagnosing diabetic nephropathy

Diabetic patients should have a specimen of urine tested for protein using a dip-stick (e.g. Albustix®) at each annual review. If protein is detected, an MSU sample should be sent to the laboratory for culture.

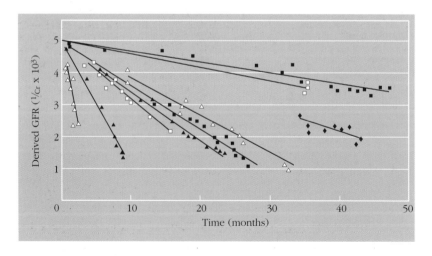

Figure 14.3 *Progressive decline in GFR with time in patients with IDDM. Reproduced with permission from Jones RH et al., 1979[4].*
Cr = serum creatinine (μmol/l).

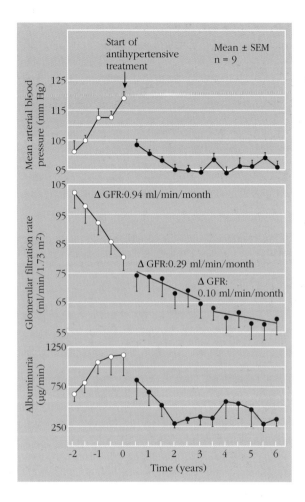

Figure 14.4 *Effect of aggressive antihypertensive treatment on renal function in patients with IDDM and nephropathy. Reproduced with permission from Parving HH et al., 1987[5].*

If a UTI is found, it should be treated appropriately with antibiotics and then a further urine sample tested for protein.

A 24-hour urine collection should be sent to the laboratory to measure urinary protein loss. Proteinuria is not pathognomonic of diabetic nephropathy, so other possible causes need to be excluded. A full history may reveal previous renal tract disease. A full examination should be performed, including fundoscopy, abdominal palpation and prostate examination in men. Renal tract ultrasound

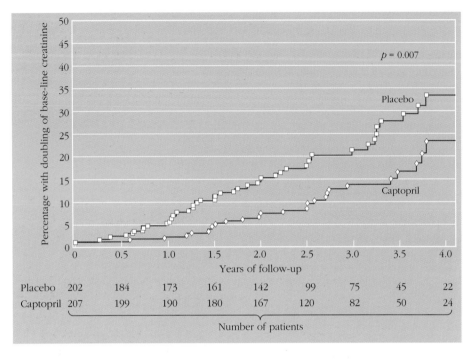

Placebo	202	184	173	161	142	99	75	45	22
Captopril	207	199	190	180	167	120	82	50	24

Number of patients

Figure 14.5 *Effect of antihypertensive treatment with the ACE inhibitor, captopril, on renal function in diabetic patients with nephropathy. Reproduced with permission from Lewis EJ et al., 1993[6].*

should also be undertaken. In general, renal biopsy is unnecessary as the diagnosis tends to be clear-cut on clinical grounds. However, the presence of IDDM for less than 10 years or the absence of diabetic retinopathy would be an indication for renal biopsy, if no other cause for renal disease were found.

Management of patients with persistent proteinuria

Any diabetic patient with proteinuria should be referred to the hospital diabetes specialist for assessment and formulation of a management plan. In many cases, a shared approach to care is valuable. The patient requires a complete explanation, including the potential gravity of the prognosis.

Management strategies involve:

- aggressive blood pressure control with treatment including an ACE inhibitor (Figure 14.5)[6]; target BP, less than 140/90 if under 50 years of age, and 150/90 if 50 years or over
- low protein diet when serum creatinine exceeds 200 μmol/l
- optimization of glycaemic control
- treatment of hyperlipidaemia
- regular review to detect other diabetic and macrovascular complications
- early referral to a nephrologist for assessment for renal replacement therapy (i.e. dialysis and/or renal transplantation).

Diabetes, blindness or amputation are not contraindications for renal replacement therapy.

Prevention of diabetic nephropathy

Early detection of microalbuminuria and its treatment may prevent or delay the progression to renal impairment. Good glycaemic control was shown in the Diabetes Control and Complications Trial to reduce the risk of developing nephropathy. There is also some evidence for a threshold level of glycaemic control above which nephropathy becomes more likely[7] (see page 15).

Other manifestations of diabetic renal disease

UTI

UTIs are common in diabetic patients, though those with good glycaemic control are no more susceptible than the general population. A UTI is likely to lead to deterioration in glycaemic control. This contributes to the patient's inability to fight the infection and the vicious circle of deteriorating control and worsening infection. Recurrent UTIs can be a significant cause of ill health and poor control, and they should be treated with a prophylactic dose of antibiotic at night (e.g. trimethoprim, 100 mg) for 6–12 months.

Autonomic neuropathy and the bladder

Decreased sensation in the bladder leads to progressive difficulty with bladder emptying and increasing bladder size. The patient may be unaware of the problem, which tends to be complicated by UTIs. Referral to a urologist is appropriate.

Renal papillary necrosis

This condition, which seldom occurs in non-diabetic people, may present acutely with loin pain, fever and malaise, though it is now recognized to be more indolent in some patients than others. Recurrent UTIs render patients, particularly women, more vulnerable to this condition.

Shared care summary

■ Diabetic nephropathy is asymptomatic until end stage renal failure sets in; screening is essential for early diagnosis and treatment to reduce progression.

■ Persistent proteinuria is characteristic of diabetic nephropathy; all diabetic patients should have urine tested for protein (with Albustix®) annually.

■ Microalbuminuria – the earliest sign of diabetic renal disease – is detectable on an early morning urine sample.

■ ACE inhibitors reduce microalbuminuria even in normotensive patients.

■ Aggressive treatment of hypertension can significantly delay the progression of diabetic nephropathy. The primary care team should be actively involved in monitoring and treatment of hypertension.

■ All patients with suspected diabetic nephropathy should be referred to the hospital diabetes team.

■ Diabetic patients with renal failure should be referred early to a nephrologist for assessment for renal replacement therapy.

■ Diabetic patients with nephropathy invariably have other diabetic complications; regular screening, whether in primary or secondary care, is vital.

References

1 Gatling W. Role of microalbuminuria in diabetes care. *Hospital Update* February 1993: 105–10.

2 Hallab M, Gallois Y, Chatellier G, Rohmer V, Fressinand P, Marre M. Comparison of reduction in microalbuminuria by enalapril and hydrochlorothiazide in normotensive patients with insulin dependent diabetes. *BMJ* 1993; **306:** 175–82.

3 Sano T, Hotta N, Kawarmura T et al. Effects of long-term enalapril treatment on persistent microalbuminuria in normotensive type 2 diabetic patients: results of a 4 year prospective randomised study. *Diabet Med* 1996; **13:** 120–4.

4 Jones RH, Hayakawa M, Mackay JD, Parsons V, Watkins PJ. Progression of diabetic nephropathy. *Lancet* 1979; **i:** 1105–6.

5 Parving HH, Andersen AR, Smidt UM, Hommel E, Mathiesen ER, Svendsen PA. Effect of antihypertensive treatment on kidney function in diabetic nephropathy. *BMJ* 1987; **294:** 1443–7.

6 Lewis EJ, Hunsicker LG, Bain RP, Rohde RD, for the Collaborative Study Group. The effect of angiotensin-converting enzyme inhibition on diabetic nephropathy. *N Engl J Med* 1993; **329:** 1456–62.

7 Krolewski AS, Laffel LMB, Krolewski M, Quinn M, Warram JH. Glycosylated hemoglobin and the risk of microalbuminuria in patients with insulin-dependent diabetes mellitus. *N Engl J Med* 1995; **332:** 1251–5.

Further reading

Viberti GC, Walker JD, Pinto J. Diabetic nephropathy. In: Alberti KGMM, DeFronzo RA, Keen H, Zimmet P, eds. *International textbook of diabetes mellitus.* Chichester: John Wiley & Sons, 1992: 1267–328.

Payton CD, Boulton AJM, Jones JM. Treatment of renal failure in diabetic patients. *Hospital Update* April 1989: 249–62.

Chapter 15

Macrovascular disease, hyperlipidaemia and hypertension

The increased prevalence of circulatory disorders among diabetic patients results in increased morbidity and mortality. This chapter considers the detection, assessment and treatment of macrovascular disease, hyperlipidaemia and hypertension.

Macrovascular disease in diabetes

Macrovascular disease is the underlying cause of death for many diabetic patients. In one community study, 55% of diabetic patients died from circulatory disease, of which 84% was due to ischaemic heart disease (IHD)[1]. Compared with the general population, people with diabetes (particularly middle-aged women) have a higher mortality due to vascular disease (Figure 15.1)[1]. Both post-mortem and angiographic studies of coronary arteries have shown that diabetic patients generally have more extensive and more severe atherosclerosis than matched non-diabetic controls.

Diabetic nephropathy causes a significant increase in macrovascular disease. Renal damage increases the prevalence of hypertension and hyperlipidaemia and accelerates the development of atheroma.

Peripheral vascular disease (PVD) is also a significant problem. The Framingham study in the USA found markedly higher incidences of PVD among diabetic patients compared with the general population: three times higher in diabetic men and six times higher in diabetic women[2].

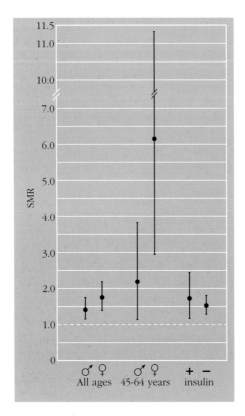

Figure 15.1 *Standardized mortality ratios (SMR; ± 95% CI) for circulatory disease in a diabetic population with follow-up for 11 years. Adapted from Walters DP et al., 1994[1] SMR = 1; no significant difference from the general population.*

Risk factors for macrovascular disease

In diabetes, the factors associated with an increased risk of macrovascular disease are:

- ■ hyperlipidaemia
- ■ hypertension
- ■ hyperinsulinaemia
- ■ diabetic nephropathy/microalbuminuria
- ■ smoking
- ■ obesity
- ■ family history of IHD.

Detection and investigation of macrovascular disease

During the annual review, diabetic patients should be questioned directly about any new symptoms, such as chest pain, breathlessness and claudication. After taking a history and carrying out an examination, appropriate investigations should be arranged. Referral, either to the diabetologist or appropriate specialist, is indicated in patients whose management is difficult or in whom further investigation, such as angiography, is required. Silent myocardial ischaemia is not uncommon in diabetic patients with coronary artery disease. This is best identified through an exercise ECG.

Treatment of macrovascular disease

Patients with macrovascular disease need review of blood pressure (BP), lipid profiles and glycaemic control with further treatment if problems are identified. Lifestyle changes, such as stopping smoking, are vital and exercise promotion is invaluable, particularly for PVD.

Antiplatelet drugs (e.g. low dose aspirin, 75–150 mg/day) are now well recognized agents for reducing the risk of myocardial infarction (MI) and thrombotic stroke among the non-diabetic population with vascular disease. Low-dose aspirin should be prescribed for all diabetic patients with macrovascular disease who have no contraindications and can tolerate it. Its use in primary prevention of vascular disease in diabetic patients is still controversial. Large prospective studies in diabetic patients are needed, though some would argue that diabetic patients with more than one risk factor for macrovascular disease should receive low-dose aspirin[3].

Full anticoagulation with drugs such as warfarin should be considered in patients at risk of arterial emboli (e.g. those in atrial fibrillation or with poor left ventricular function and a dilated heart).

Insulin treated diabetic patients with angina or post-MI can be treated with β-blockers, preferably of the cardioselective type. If loss of warning symptoms of hypoglycaemia is a problem, alternative agents (e.g. calcium channel blockers or nitrates) may be used. Patients with significant macrovascular disease should be encouraged to avoid frequent episodes of hypoglycaemia. Low blood glucose levels could be dangerous to ischaemic tissue (e.g. triggering dysrhythmias in the post-MI situation, reducing tissue viability in the ischaemic brain or limb).

MI is recognized to result in higher mortality and morbidity in diabetic patients than in comparable non-diabetic controls. People with diabetes tend to suffer larger infarcts with greater damage, which tends to cause left ventricular failure. Angiotensin converting enzyme (ACE) inhibitors are now being used routinely when heart failure is diagnosed after an MI.

Problems with blood lipids in diabetes

Lipid metabolism in diabetes is influenced by insulin deficiency, insulin resistance, glycaemic control, obesity, diet, exercise and genetic factors. The majority of patients with well controlled insulin dependent diabetes mellitus (IDDM) have normal lipid profiles. Those with hyperlipidaemia generally have poor glycaemic control, a family history of lipid problems or diabetic nephropathy. The converse is seen in patients with non-insulin dependent diabetes mellitus (NIDDM), most of whom have dyslipidaemia due to the well recognized association between hyperlipidaemia, hyperinsulinaemia and NIDDM (syndrome X)[4].

All the major lipoproteins circulating in the blood are complex molecular aggregates involving cholesterol. Low density lipoprotein (LDL) accounts for approximately 70% of circulating cholesterol and is atherogenic. Correlations between total cholesterol and coronary artery disease are almost entirely due to the LDL cholesterol concentration. High density lipoprotein (HDL) is involved in the reverse transport of cholesterol to the liver for metabolism and is cardioprotective.

Hyperlipidaemia is associated with an increased risk of macrovascular disease. Raised lipid levels may be lowered by diet and a variety of lipid lowering agents (Table 15.1)[5]. The assumption that its early treatment will reduce the progression of atheroma and, consequently, improve the long-term outcome for patients with diabetes remains to be proved. A WHO multicentre trial, the Diabetes

Table 15.1 Drugs used in the treatment of hyperlipidaemia[5]

	Statin	Fibrate	Resin	Nicotinic acid type
Examples	Simvastatin Pravastatin Fluvastatin	Bezafibrate Ciprofibrate Fenofibrate Gemfibrozil	Cholestyramine Colestipol	Acipimox
Mode of action	↓ HMG-CoA reductase	↑ Adipose lipoprotein lipase	Anion exchange resin. Binds bile acids in GI tract	↓ VLDL synthesis
Effect	TC ↓ 25–30% HDL-C ↑ 8–10% TG ↓ 5–15%	TC ↓ 5–30% HDL ↑ 15–25% TG ↓ 30%	TC ↓ 15–30% TG ↑ 5–15%	TC ↓ 5–15% TG ↓ 15–30%
Contraindications	Liver disease, porphyria, pregnancy or breast-feeding	Gall bladder disease, severe liver or renal impairment, pregnancy or breast-feeding	Biliary obstruction	Peptic ulcer, pregnancy
Adverse events	GI upset, headache, hepatitis (check LFTs), myositis (check CPK)	GI upset, hair loss, headache, myositis (check CPK)	Bleeding tendency, GI upset	Flushing, itching and rash, GI upset
Interactions	Cyclosporin, fibrates, warfarin	OHAs, statins, warfarin	Acarbose, digoxin and diuretics, paracetamol, thyroxine, vancomycin, warfarin	

CPK = creatine phosphokinase; GI = gastrointestinal; HDL-C = high-density lipoprotein cholesterol; HMG-CoA = hydroxymethylglutaryl coenzyme A; LFTs = liver function tests; OHA = oral hypoglycaemic agents; TC = total cholesterol; TG = triglyceride; VLDL = very low density lipoproteins.

Atherosclerosis Intervention Study (DAIS), has specifically enrolled diabetic patients and will compare fenofibrate treatment with placebo. This study will not be completed for at least 3 years.

Two large trials (the West of Scotland study[6], a primary prevention study, and the 4S study[7], a secondary prevention study) have recently been carried out with statins, which inhibit hydroxymethylglutaryl coenzyme A reductase, the rate limiting enzyme in the hepatic production of cholesterol. These trials resulted in a 20–30% reduction in all deaths in patients treated with the lipid lowering agents compared with placebo; a 30% reduction in non-fatal MIs and a 37% reduction in the need for coronary revascularization procedures were also noted. Subgroup analysis has shown that the benefit for diabetic patients receiving active treatment was greater than for the group as a whole (Table 15.2)[8]. These trial results have led to a far more active approach to the management of hyperlipidaemia. Interestingly, both trials showed a significant reduction in mortality within 2 years of treatment, suggesting that statins may act through other mechanisms, such as plaque stabilization or local endothelial dependent vasorelaxation, as well as by the significant lowering of serum cholesterol levels.

Table 15.2 Reduction in major coronary events with simvastatin treatment (the 4S trial[8])

	Placebo treatment		Simvastatin treatment		Relative risk (95% CI)
	Total number	Number with coronary event	Total number	Number with coronary event	
Diabetes	92	44 (45%)	105	24 (23%)	0.45 (0.27–0.74)
No diabetes	2126	578 (27%)	2116	407 (19%)	0.68 (0.60–0.77)

Selection criteria for the trial: men and women aged 35–70 years with a history of angina or MI and with serum total cholesterol 5.5–8.0 mmol/l and triglyceride < 2.5 mmol/l.

The lipid profile

When lipid determinations are requested, many laboratories provide only an initial screen of cholesterol and triglyceride (TG) concentrations, which is inadequate for diabetic patients (Figure 15.2; RD Hill, unpublished data). Screening and monitoring lipid levels in diabetic patients should include HDL-cholesterol as well as total cholesterol and TG concentrations.

Fasting blood samples are preferred for lipid analysis as TG levels (though not cholesterol) vary according to food intake. Obtaining blood samples after a minimum of 10 hours' fasting may be difficult or even dangerous in insulin treated patients because of the risk of hypoglycaemia. A random sample is a possible solution. If the TG concentration is satisfactory when non-fasting, this fact is reassuring. However, the LDL result is likely to be inaccurate on a non-fasting sample, as LDL (being difficult to measure directly) is usually calculated from other values, including TG.

Detection and assessment of hyperlipidaemia

A system for screening diabetic patients for hyperlipidaemia is outlined in Figure 15.3. Safe lipid levels in diabetic patients are still far from clear and thresholds for drug treatment are being progressively lowered, particularly for those with evidence of macrovascular disease.

Assessment of the diabetic patient with hyperlipidaemia

Assessment and management of hyperlipidaemia is outlined in Figure 15.4. Review of current therapy may enable withdrawal or dose reduction of any drugs liable to affect blood lipids adversely (e.g. thiazide diuretics, β-blockers, steroids, cyclosporin, oral contraceptives, retinoids). Alternative causes of secondary hyperlipidaemia (e.g. hypothyroidism, renal failure, liver disease, excessive alcohol intake) need to be excluded.

Poor glycaemic control leads to hypertriglyceridaemia and, to a lesser extent, raised cholesterol. Efforts should be made to optimize control before reviewing the lipids again. If, despite best efforts,

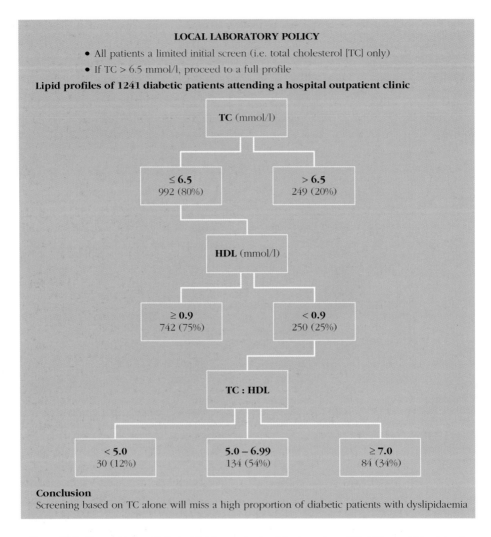

LOCAL LABORATORY POLICY
- All patients a limited initial screen (i.e. total cholesterol [TC] only)
- If TC > 6.5 mmol/l, proceed to a full profile

Lipid profiles of 1241 diabetic patients attending a hospital outpatient clinic

TC (mmol/l)

≤ 6.5
992 (80%)

> 6.5
249 (20%)

HDL (mmol/l)

≥ 0.9
742 (75%)

< 0.9
250 (25%)

TC : HDL

< 5.0
30 (12%)

5.0 – 6.99
134 (54%)

≥ 7.0
84 (34%)

Conclusion
Screening based on TC alone will miss a high proportion of diabetic patients with dyslipidaemia

Figure 15.2 *The problem with limited lipid screening in diabetic patients (RD Hill, unpublished data).*

glycaemic control is difficult to improve, specific therapy should be aimed at the hyperlipidaemia. Treatment with a fibrate may also benefit glycaemic control.

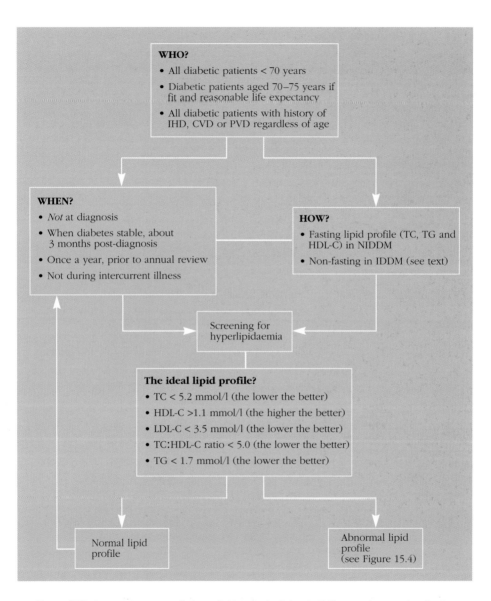

Figure 15.3 *A screening system for hyperlipidaemia in diabetes. CVD = cerebrovascular disease; TG = triglyceride; TC = total cholesterol; HDL-C = HDL cholesterol; LDL-C = LDL cholesterol.*

A poor lipid profile should be reviewed in the light of other risk factors for macrovascular disease and evidence for existing macrovascular disease.

Management of hyperlipidaemia

The initial management (Figure 15.4) should be aimed at lifestyle changes, including a low-fat diet, weight reduction, lowering alcohol intake and stopping smoking. All diabetic patients with lipid problems benefit from review by a dietitian (see Chapter 5). Increasing regular physical activity can improve the lipid profile by raising the serum HDL level. In post-menopausal women, the introduction of hormone replacement therapy leads to an improved lipid profile as LDL cholesterol is reduced and HDL cholesterol is raised. Oral oestrogen may aggravate hypertriglyceridaemia, but oestrogen taken transdermally does not have this effect.

After a 3–6-month trial of diet and lifestyle changes, the lipid profile should be reassessed. If the trend is towards improvement and the disturbance is only mild, continuation of the lifestyle changes may be sufficient. Threshold lipid levels for the introduction of lipid lowering agents are given in Figure 15.4. It is difficult to give any hard and fast rules concerning age and the introduction of drug therapy for hyperlipidaemia. Each patient should be considered according to risks and life expectancy.

Threshold lipid levels for treating those with established macrovascular disease are lower than those for patients with risk factors alone. The significant reduction in morbidity and mortality from cardiovascular disease in the West of Scotland Study[6] and the 4S trial[7] have reinforced the use of the statins, which impressively reduce cholesterol levels. Fibrates, which have their strongest effect on reducing TG levels, have yet to show such significant improvements in clinical outcome in longer-term trials. Thus, on current evidence, patients with coronary artery disease (or a high risk of developing it) should probably be treated with a statin as first-line therapy, if total serum cholesterol is above 5.5 mmol/l.

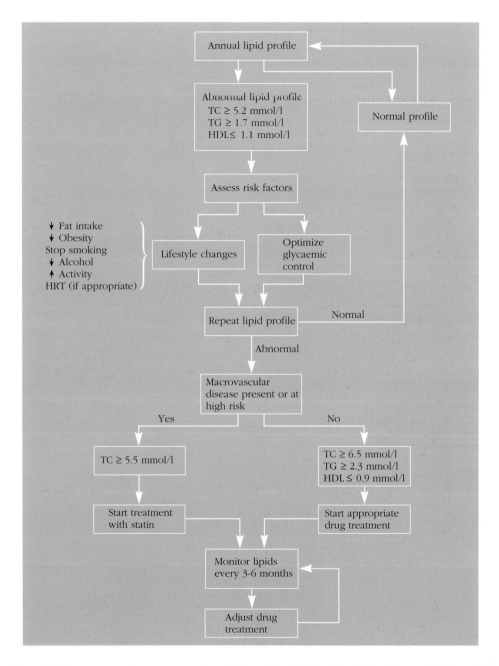

Figure 15.4 *Assessment and management of hyperlipidaemia in diabetic patients. Abbreviations as for Figure 15.3.*

The majority of diabetic patients have a mixed hyperlipidaemia picture with considerable hypertriglyceridaemia and thus, first-line treatment is generally a fibrate. If after 3–6 months of diet and drug therapy, the lipid profile is still significantly deranged, combination drug therapy may be considered. Referral for specialist evaluation, either by the diabetologist or at a lipid clinic, is valuable at this stage.

Hypertension

Hypertension is common among patients with NIDDM in whom the prevalence is a remarkable 25–40%. Indeed, hypertension may be present prior to diagnosis of diabetes. By contrast, hypertension is uncommon in IDDM except when associated with microalbuminuria or diabetic nephropathy and in a few patients with essential hypertension, when a family history is often found. The UKPDS data (Figure 15.5)[9] suggest that hypertension is underdiagnosed and undertreated in all age groups, but particularly among younger patients. Patients with NIDDM often have the combination of obesity, hyperinsulinaemia and hyperlipidaemia known as 'syndrome X'[4] and

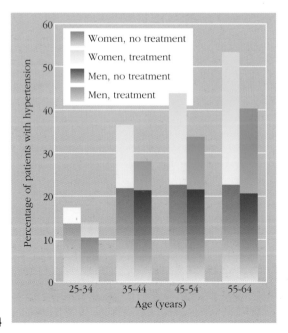

Figure 15.5 *Prevalence of hypertension (defined as BP ≥ 160/90) in NIDDM at diagnosis among those either receiving or not receiving antihypertensive treatment. Data from the UK Prospective Diabetes Study[9].*

they are at increased risk of developing IHD and other macrovascular complications. Causes of secondary hypertension, though unusual, should also be considered and investigated appropriately.

The benefits of treating patients with diabetes for hypertension are considerable, as these patients are at increased risk of stroke, renal disease and heart failure. Certainly, the age-adjusted mortality rises more dramatically with systolic BP in diabetic patents than in the non-diabetic population (Figure 15.6). Treatment of hypertension in the general population is now well recognized to reduce the risk of cerebrovascular and cardiovascular disease and to delay the progression of renal failure. Diabetic microvascular complications, such as retinopathy and nephropathy, progress more rapidly in uncontrolled hypertension.

Definition of hypertension

Hypertension is generally diagnosed when the BP is consistently greater than 160/90. Isolated systolic hypertension requires treatment

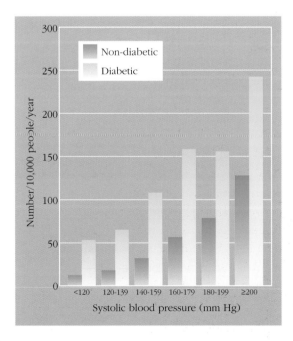

Figure 15.6 Age-adjusted 10-year mortality by systolic blood pressure and history of diabetes (the MRFIT screened cohort). Adapted form Stanilev J et al.[10].

as much as diastolic hypertension. The conventional definition of hypertension may be inadequate in some groups of diabetic patients, particularly teenagers, young adults and those with diabetic complications. BP greater than 140/90 is significant in those aged under 40 and in those with complications. Even lower cut-off levels may be required in adolescents. *All diabetic patients should have annual BP measurements* and if greater than 140/90, more frequent monitoring is necessary.

Blood pressure measurement

In the UK, British Hypertension Society guidelines[11] are appropriate for BP measurement. Two measurements should be taken at each visit with the patient seated and rested. Lying and standing measurements are necessary in the elderly and in diabetic hypertensive patients as postural hypotension is common.

Management of hypertension

Basic investigations in diabetic hypertensive patients: urine should be tested for protein and blood and a specimen sent for microscopy and culture. Plasma urea and electrolytes and serum creatinine should be determined. Further investigations might include an ultrasound scan of the renal tract, an echocardiogram, a chest radiograph, and microalbuminuria screen.

Primary care is the ideal setting for assessing, managing and monitoring hypertension. Monitoring BP levels can be undertaken by the practice nurse, while the doctor may review the results at intervals. Attendance at hospital is usually associated with some degree of anxiety, which is likely to lead to raised BP — sometimes referred to as 'white coat hypertension'. This phenomenon must be taken into account, as it can lead to overtreatment and resultant adverse events. Some patients like to monitor their own BP at home, and these results can be very useful. Ambulatory monitoring is becoming increasingly available in general practice and can help to avoid 'white coat hypertension'.

Table 15.3 Acceptable blood pressure targets*

Age (years)	Systolic (mmHg)	Diastolic (mmHg)
< 50	140	< 90
50–65	150	90
> 65	160	90

*These are general guidelines. Individual patient targets should be developed after considering all factors.

Approaches to management: treatment should be tailored to the individual and BP gradually lowered over a period of weeks, particularly in the elderly. Acceptable BP targets are given in Table 15.3. Drug regimens should be as simple as possible, as most patients are already taking other medication, and good compliance is important to successful BP control. As with all aspects of diabetes management, explanation and education of the patient about the importance of treating hypertension is essential. Recording the results of BP measurements in the patients' record books may promote their involvement.

Lifestyle changes should be the first line of management for patients with mild or borderline hypertension. Weight loss, and reduction of salt intake and alcohol consumption can modestly lower BP. Combining these changes with an increase in physical activity will help to improve general fitness and may be beneficial to the serum lipid profile.

Drug treatment: antihypertensive agents (Table 15.4) should be selected with care for diabetic patients. ACE inhibitors should be considered as first choice agents, especially in patients with nephropathy. If these are contraindicated or poorly tolerated, calcium channel blockers are a suitable alternative. A new category of drug,

Table 15.4 Antihypertensive agents

	ACE inhibitors	Calcium channel blockers	α-blockers	Thiazide diuretics	β-blockers	Angiotensin II receptor antagonists
Use in diabetic patients	First line	First line	Second line	Seldom indicated	Useful in angina and CAD. Use cardioselective	Consider if dry cough with ACE inhibitor
Examples	Enalapril Lisinopril Ramipril	Amlodipine Lacidipine Nifedipine	Doxazosin	Bendrofluazide	Atenolol Metoproplol Bisoprolol	Losartan
Benefits	Reduce proteinuria and conserve renal function in nephropathy. Reduce LV hypertrophy. Beneficial in heart failure	Reduce LV hypertrophy. More effective in Afro-Caribbeans	Beneficial in impotence?	Inexpensive	Useful in patients with angina	Similar to ACE inhibitors but no dry cough
Cautions	Avoid in pregnancy. Beware first dose hypotension. Avoid with potassium-sparing diuretics. Provokes hyperkalaemia in renal impairment. Avoid with renal artery stenosis. Check renal function 2 weeks after starting treatment	Avoid in pregnancy. Avoid nifedipine in heart failure. Reduce dose if liver impairment	Beware first dose postural hypotension. Avoid in autonomic neuropathy	Avoid in pregnancy. Aggravates diabetes and gout. Use with care if renal failure or hepatic impairment	Avoid in PVD. Avoid in asthma or heart failure. Mask hypoglycaemic symptoms. Reduce dose if renal impairment	See ACE inhibitors

Significant adverse events	Dry cough, angioedema and urticaria, symptom complex of fever, rash, vasculitis, myalgia and arthralgia	Headache, flushing, oedema, tachycardia, gum hyperplasia	Postural hypotension, headache, oedema	Postural hypotension, hypokalaemia, impotence	Bradycardia, fatigue, sleep disturbance, cold extremities, impotence, weight gain	Rash, hypotension, hyperkalaemia, liver function changes
Effect on lipids	None	None	May improve lipid profile	Deterioration in lipid profile	Deterioration in lipid profile, though not with bisoprolol	None
Effect on glucose tolerance	None	None	None	Impaired	Possibly impaired	None
Significant interactions	Alcohol, antidepressants, allopurinol, lithium, levodopa, NSAIDs	Anti-convulsants, β-blockers, cyclosporin, digoxin	Alcohol, anti-depressants, levodopa	Antidepressants, lithium	Alcohol, calcium channel blockers	As for ACE inhibitors

ACE = angiotensin converting enzyme; CaD = coronary artery disease; LV = left ventricular; NSAIDs = non-steroidal anti-inflammatory drugs; PVD = peripheral vascular disease.

the angiotensin II receptor antagonist, losartan, has recently become available and would be suitable for patients developing cough as a side-effect of an ACE inhibitor.

Monotherapy may not adequately control hypertension, so combination treatment is often necessary. Calcium channel blockers or α-blockers combine well with ACE inhibitors. Diuretics are recognized to potentiate the hypotensive action of ACE inhibitors, but a loop diuretic (e.g. frusemide) should be used. Thiazide diuretics should be avoided because of their adverse effect on glucose tolerance and lipid profiles. Potassium sparing diuretics (e.g. amiloride) can lead to hyperkalaemia with ACE inhibitors.

Triple therapy may be required for some patients; referral to the diabetologist may be useful if this is the case. Overall, the choice of additional drug depends on the individual patient and on other concomitant disease, such as IHD, heart failure or autonomic neuropathy. Optimal BP control, which should be the aim of treatment, will often have to be balanced by side-effects of therapy.

Shared care summary

■ Macrovascular disease accounts for significant morbidity and mortality in diabetic patients.

■ The identification and modification of risk factors for macrovascular disease in diabetic patients should lead to improved outcome.

■ Treatment of macrovascular disease should include antiplatelet therapy, such as low-dose aspirin.

■ Referral for further investigation and treatment should be considered in all patients with macrovascular disease.

■ Diabetic patients should have a lipid profile check annually, and those with hyperlipidaemia should be treated, particularly if macrovascular disease is also present.

■ Lifestyle changes represent first-line therapy for hyperlipidaemia; if they are unsuccessful or insufficient, drug therapy should be considered.

■ Hypertension is associated with increased morbidity and mortality in diabetic patients and should be diagnosed and treated.

■ Primary care is the ideal setting for monitoring and treating hypertension. Thresholds for treatment of hypertension are lower in diabetic patients, particularly those with complications, than in the general population.

■ Antihypertensive agents need to be selected with care for diabetic patients.

References

1 Walters DP, Gatling W, Houston AC, Mullee MA, Julious SA, Hill RD. Mortality in diabetic subjects: an eleven-year follow-up of a community-based population. *Diabet Med* 1994; **11:** 968–73.

2 Kannel WB, McGee DL. Diabetes and glucose tolerance as risk factors for cardiovascular disease: the Framingham study. *Diabetes Care* 1979; **2:** 120–6.

3 Yudkin JS. Which diabetic patients should be taking aspirin? *BMJ* 1995; **311:** 641–2.

4 Reaven GM. Role of insulin resistance in human disease. *Diabetes* 1988; **37:** 1595–607.

5 O'Connor P, Feely J, Shepherd J. Lipid lowering drugs. *BMJ* 1990; **300:** 667–72.

6 Shepherd J, Cobb SM, Ford I *et al.* for the West of Scotland Coronary Prevention Study Group. Prevention of coronary heart disease with pravastatin in men with hypercholesterolemia. *N Engl J Med* 1995; **333:** 1301–7.

7 Scandinavian Simvastatin Survival Study Group. Randomised trial of cholesterol lowering in 4444 patients with coronary heart disease: the Scandinavian Simvastatin Survival Study (4S). *Lancet* 1994; **344:** 1383–9.

8 Kjekshus J, Pedersen TR, for the Scandinavian Simvastatin Survival Study Group. Reducing the risk of coronary events: evidence from the Scandinavian Simvastatin Survival Study (4S). *Am J Cardiol* 1995; **76:** 64–8C.

9 The Hypertension in Diabetes Study Group. Hypertension in diabetes study (HDS): 1. Prevalence of hypertension in newly presenting type 2 diabetic patients and the association with risk factors for cardiovascular and diabetic complications. *J Hypertens* 1993; **11:** 309–17.

10 Stanilev J, Vaccaroo O, Neaton JD, Wentworth D, for the Multiple Risk Factor Intervention Trial Research Group. Diabetes, other risk factors, and 12-year cardiovascular mortality for men screened in the Multiple Risk Factor Intervention Trial. *Diabetes Care* 1993; **16:** 434–44.

11 British Hypertension Society. Management guidelines in essential hypertension: report of the second working party of the British Hypertension Society. *BMJ* 1993; **306:** 983–7.

Further reading

Dean JD, Durrington PN. Treatment of dyslipoproteinaemia in diabetes mellitus. *Diabet Med* 1996; **13:** 297–312.

Durrington PN. Prevention of macrovascular disease: absolute proof or absolute risk? *Diabet Med* 1995; **12:** 561–2.

European Atherosclerosis Society. Prevention of coronary heart disease — scientific background and new clinical guidelines. *Nutr Metab Cardiovasc Dis* 1992; **2:** 113–56.

Feher MD. *Hypertension and diabetes mellitus*. London: Martin Dunitz, 1993.

Reckless JPD. *Diabetes and lipids*. London: Martin Dunitz, 1994.

Shaper AG, Perry IJ. Screening people with diabetes for risk of coronary heart disease in general practice. *Practical Diabetes* 1994; **11:** 228–31.

Blood pressure and diabetes: everyone's concern. A Working Party Report. Chineham, Hampshire, UK: RRAssoc, 1994.

Chapter 16

Diabetic neuropathy

Hyperglycaemia has a significant effect on nerve function and structure. Although the earliest manifestations may be detected only by electrophysiological studies, nerve function may become so severely disordered that neuropathic diabetic foot disease develops or sudden death occurs due to autonomic neuropathy. The importance of diabetic neuropathy is related, therefore, to the increase in morbidity and mortality it produces. Regular screening and early detection of neuropathy are imperative for the prevention of serious consequences.

In this chapter, diabetic neuropathy is defined and classified, and the various types are considered from the standpoint of diagnosis, referral and treatment. Effective treatment is difficult, and the pivotal role of good glycaemic control in the prevention of neuropathy is emphasized throughout.

Prevalence and incidence figures for diabetic neuropathy are difficult to obtain because neuropathy has no precise definition. If a purely electrophysiological definition is used, and the criterion for diagnosis is slowed nerve conduction, then 100% of diabetic patients have neuropathy. Young et al.[1], using different criteria, found a prevalence of 28.3% with a positive correlation with age and duration of diabetes.

Since no part of the peripheral nervous system escapes the effects of hyperglycaemia, the manifestations of diabetic neuropathy vary according to the particular type of nerve predominantly affected.

Classification and definitions of diabetic neuropathy

In an attempt to clarify a complex situation, the various types of diabetic neuropathy have been classified as follows:

- electrophysiological neuropathy
- subjective neuropathy
- objective neuropathy
- autonomic neuropathy.

Electrophysiological neuropathy: this condition is demonstrable only by nerve conduction studies. It is not associated with any signs or symptoms and is usually reversible with good glycaemic control over a period of a few months.

Subjective neuropathy may be defined as neuropathy associated with dysaesthesia giving rise to symptoms in the absence of any physical signs. This type of neuropathy is also generally reversible with good glycaemic control.

Objective neuropathy: in this condition, the patient not only has symptoms suggesting neuropathy, but there are also demonstrable physical signs and electrophysiological changes. Focal or multifocal neuropathy (affecting either a single nerve trunk or several different nerve trunks) is almost certainly caused by vascular events. It is typified by the cranial neuropathies (e.g. third nerve palsy (Figure 16.1) or sixth nerve palsy), thoraco-abdominal neuropathies (see page 265), focal limb neuropathies and diabetic amyotrophy. Recovery may occur over a period of 3 months to 2 years.

The commonest type of neuropathy is symmetrical sensorimotor polyneuropathy. This is the typical diabetic peripheral neuropathy affecting the legs and feet (see page 268). A less common form of symmetrical neuropathy is proximal lower limb motor neuropathy. The patient may recover but only slowly over 6–12 months.

Diabetic amyotrophy has an acute onset. There is often considerable pain in the affected muscles (usually the thighs), and the

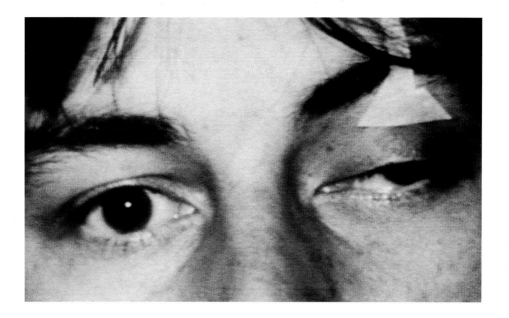

Figure 16.1 *Patient with third nerve palsy.*

onset is often associated with weight loss and preceded by a period of poor glycaemic control.

Autonomic neuropathy (see page 208): the effects of damage to the autonomic nervous system are widespread and, in the early stages, asymptomatic.

Aetiology of neuropathy
Neuropathy has a multifactorial aetiology, though metabolic and vascular changes predominate. Metabolic changes are governed by hyperglycaemia, and the vascular changes are similar to other microangiopathies affecting the eye and the kidneys (see Chapters 13 and 14).

Affected nerves show axonal degeneration and regeneration. The myelin sheath disappears in segments of the nerves and is later reconstructed. The blood vessels supplying the nerves show closure and thrombosis, which causes neuronal ischaemia and dysfunction. The metabolic changes involved in the aetiology of neuropathy include abnormalities of sorbitol metabolism and other pathways (Figure 16.2).

Diagnosis and investigation

As neuropathy may be either asymptomatic or associated with only minimal or nonspecific symptoms, its presence needs to be actively sought at each patient's annual review (see Chapter 11). Detection is particularly important, despite the difficulty of treating or reversing established neuropathy; much can be gained by educating the patient in the prevention of future problems.

Diagnosis of neuropathy can be reached by taking a careful history and carrying out a systematic, thorough, clinical examination.

Patients may complain of numbness, tingling and pain in the feet, which is generally worse in bed at night. The pain may have the peculiar characteristics of a piercing or shooting pain. Such pain may be present even in a foot that has lost pain sensation on formal testing.

The various modalities of nerve function should be tested as follows:

- light touch (by touching not stroking the skin)
- pain sensation
- vibration sense
- knee and ankle reflexes.

Exclusion of other treatable causes of peripheral neuropathy (e.g. vitamin B_{12} or folate deficiency) is important, and a history of alcohol intake should be sought. If the diagnosis is in doubt, nerve conduction studies should be requested. Referral to the diabetologist is a sensible step.

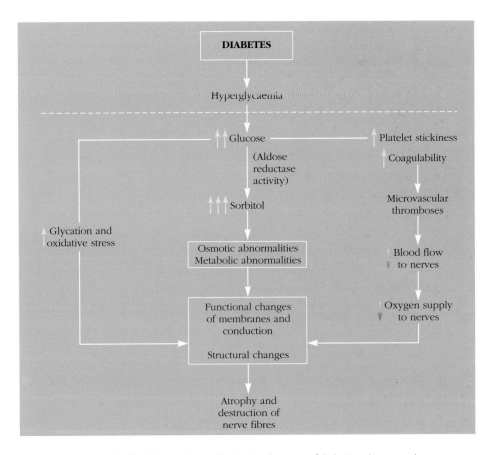

Figure 16.2 *Possible mechanism for the development of diabetic polyneuropathy.*

Treatment of neuropathy

As yet, there is no known treatment for diabetic neuropathy, so prevention should be the primary objective. For all types of diabetic neuropathy, maintenance of good glycaemic control is the best method of prevention.

Theoretically, an aldose reductase inhibitor may help to prevent or relieve neuropathy by inhibiting sorbitol production in the nerves, but there is no firm evidence of the effectiveness of this approach to date.

Evening primrose oil, a rich source of γ-linolenic acid, production of which is essential for healthy nerve function, is sometimes given to patients with diabetic neuropathy[2]. When pain is the predominant symptom, simple analgesics (e.g. paracetamol, codeine) should be tried first. Unfortunately, neuropathic pain is often unresponsive to analgesics, even opiates. Tricyclic antidepressants (e.g. amitryptyline, imipramine) may be helpful when taken at night, as they raise the pain threshold, promote sleep and improve the accompanying depression. Carbamazepine is a valuable alternative for raising the pain threshold. It should be carefully explained to the patient that neither carbamazepine nor tricyclic antidepressants relieve the pain completely, but they can make it more tolerable (see page 266).

Good glycaemic control has been shown to be the most important factor in shortening the recovery time for patients with amyotrophy. Patients with non-insulin dependent diabetes mellitus (NIDDM) may require conversion to insulin therapy in order to optimize glycaemic control and promote recovery from painful neuropathy.

On the whole, patients need support and encouragement. For most of them, the distressing symptoms are not permanent and the situation usually improves over a period of 3 months to 2 years, through either regeneration or death of the nerves concerned.

When to refer

All patients with somatosensory neuropathy affecting the legs should be referred. These patients are at great risk of the development of diabetic foot disease and need assessment by an expert. If necessary, protective footwear should be prescribed (see Chapter 17).

Autonomic neuropathy

The autonomic nervous system plays an important integrating role and extends to all parts of the body. It is not surprising, therefore, that damage to this part of the nervous system has widespread effects, which include abnormalities of:

- heart rate control
- pupilo-motor function
- gastrointestinal motility
- genito-urinary function
- vasomotor control.

Autonomic neuropathy may be either symptomatic or asymptomatic. Patients may have one or more of the symptoms listed in Table 16.1. Patients with autonomic neuropathy are prone to sudden death of unknown cause (possibly cardiovascular and arrhythmic in origin). In patients with advanced diabetic autonomic neuropathy, co-existent nephropathy, retinopathy and peripheral neuropathy are common. Autonomic neuropathy gives rise to medial calcification of blood vessels with altered blood flow and, for example, an altered ankle brachial pressure index (see page 222).

In clinical practice, the simplest tests for autonomic neuropathy are to look for variability of the pulse rate with inspiration and expiration and to measure the blood pressure in both lying and standing positions.

Treatment of autonomic neuropathy

Again, prevention is better than cure, so good glycaemic control is essential. Treatment of established autonomic neuropathy is difficult and

Table 16.1 Symptoms of autonomic neuropathy

- Dizziness on standing, due to postural hypotension
- Nocturnal diarrhoea
- Vomiting, due to gastric stasis
- Constipation
- Abnormal sweating (often gustatory)
- Impotence (see page 210)

requires caution. Certain drugs, which exacerbate postural hypotension, should be avoided; these include antihypertensive agents, diuretics, tricyclic antidepressants, nitrates and phenothiazines. Patients with suspected autonomic neuropathy should be referred to a diabetic specialist for further investigation, assessment and treatment.

Impotence in diabetes

Impotence has been reported to affect about 40% of diabetic men[3]. It is not solely a neuropathic complication but tends to be multifactorial. The factors involved include neurological damage (to peripheral and autonomic nerves), vascular disease, hormonal and psychological problems. Each patient should be assessed with a full history and examination. A hormone profile (testosterone, prolactin, luteinizing hormone and follicle stimulating hormone) should be requested.

A range of treatment options are now available, and any patient considering active treatment should be referred with his partner either to a diabetologist or to a urologist, depending on local service provision. Once testosterone deficiency has been excluded, the following options require consideration:

- a vacuum device
- intracavernosal injection of adprostadil (Caverject®) or papaverine
- a surgical penile implant.

Adprostadil is now widely used, as many patients cope with the self-injection technique (Figure 16.3). Referral for training in self injection by a doctor with appropriate expertise is advisable in order to avoid the occurrence of complications.

A recent study obtained encouraging results with a cream applied to the penis[4]. The cream contained three different vasodilators and in the laboratory increased penile arterial flow significantly. However, in a mixed group of patients, those with a suspected psychogenic origin of erectile dysfunction showed a better response.

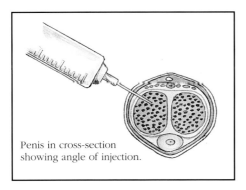

Penis in cross-section showing angle of injection.

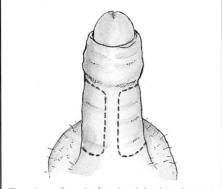

Top view of penis showing injection site area.

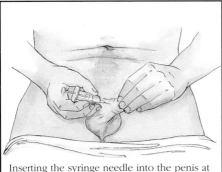

Inserting the syringe needle into the penis at injection site.

Figure 16.3 *Intracavernosal injection with adprostadil or papaverine to relax the smooth muscle of the corpora cavernosa and allow them to fill with blood, resulting in erection.*

Shared care summary

■ Neuropathy is a common complication of diabetes with potentially serious consequences. It may be avoided by the maintenance of good glycaemic control.

■ Annual screening for neuropathy is essential for its early detection.

■ As established neuropathy can be difficult to treat, patients should be referred to a diabetologist for assessment.

■ Treatment of neuropathy involves the achievement of excellent glycaemic control, plus analgesics and possibly other drugs, such as tricyclic antidepressants or carbamazepine, to help relieve pain.

■ Symptoms of painful neuropathy generally improve over a period of 3 months to 2 years.

■ Patients with neuropathy benefit from regular support from the primary care team.

■ Neuropathy may cause impotence in diabetic men. Referral to the relevant specialist for assessment and treatment is appropriate.

References

1 Young MS, Boulton AJM, McLeod AF, Williams DDR, Sonksen PH. A multicentre study of the prevalence of diabetic peripheral neuropathy in the UK hospital clinic population. *Diabetologia* 1993; **36:** 150–4.

2 Jamal GA, Carmichael H. The effect of γ-linolenic acid on human diabetic peripheral neuropathy. A double-blind, placebo-controlled trial. *Diabet Med* 1990; **7:** 319–23.

3 McCulloch DK, Campbell IW, Wu FC, Prescott RJ, Clarke BF. The prevalence of diabetic impotence. *Diabetologia* 1980; **18:** 279–83.

4 Gomaa A, Shalaby M, Osman M *et al.* Topical treatment of erectile dysfunction: randomised double blind placebo controlled trial of cream containing aminophylline, isosorbide dinitrate and co-dergocrine mesylate. *BMJ* 1996; **312:** 1512–5

Further reading

Wires PG. Erectile impotence in diabetic men: aetiology, investigation and management. *Diabet Med* 1992; **9:** 888–92.

Chapter 17

Diabetic foot disease

In diabetic foot disease, various pathological processes conspire to inflict such tissue damage that amputation may eventually be necessary. The burden of suffering and cost is enormous. In the USA, 5–15% of all patients with diabetes require some form of amputation. In the UK, the prevalence of amputation among diabetic patients over 20 years of age is 3%, and for ulceration, the prevalence is 7%. Such a degree of morbidity clearly has a large economic impact.

This chapter covers the risk factors for diabetic foot disease and its management. It emphasizes the importance of early identification of the 'at risk' patient and explains how an ulcer prevention programme can significantly reduce the incidence of foot ulcers.

Conditions predisposing to diabetic foot disease

The aetiology of diabetic foot disease is multifactorial and complex. The contributory factors are outlined in Figure 17.1.

High-risk patients

Patients with diabetes who are most likely to develop diabetic foot disease are characterized by having some or all of the following risk factors:

- neuropathy
- peripheral vascular disease (PVD)

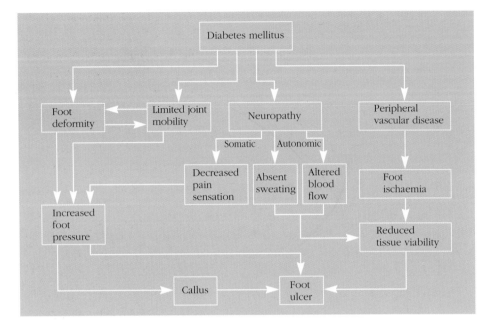

Figure 17.1 *Factors contributing to diabetic foot disease.*

- foot deformity
- infection (either fungal or bacterial)
- poor grasp of essential foot care
- poor hygiene
- smoking (either present or past)
- poor glycaemic control
- oedema of the foot
- an age of 65 years or more
- obesity
- macrovascular disease (elsewhere in the body)
- dyslipidaemia.

Neuropathic ulceration

In the neuropathic foot, the reduction in pain and temperature appreciation results in unperceived mechanical, thermal or chemical trauma. In addition, autonomic neuropathy alters haemodynamics and blood flow distribution.

In the healthy foot, the pressure generated by the weight of the body is distributed over the foot without any regions of very high pressure. However, in the deformed foot, high pressure areas develop and produce vertical and shearing stresses, which mechanically traumatize the tissues. High pressure areas occur particularly under the metatarsal heads, on the tips of the toes, and on the heel. Callus formation, which may lead to ulceration (Figure 17.2; and see page 268), raises suspicions of the existence of high pressure areas.

Thermal trauma usually occurs because of careless use of hot water bottles, electric fires or radiators. Chemical trauma to the neuropathic foot is most commonly caused by the inappropriate use of corn plasters (salicylic acid).

Ischaemic ulceration and gangrene

Trauma, which is often minor, is the initiating event in the development of ulceration or gangrene. The trauma may have its origin in pressure exerted by shoes, by sock seams, by inexpert nail cutting, or by thermal or chemical damage.

There may be a history of intermittent claudication or pain at rest. The severity of pain depends on the degree of co-existent neuropathy.

Clinical examination reveals a cold, often blue, foot with poor capillary circulation. Ulcers (Figure 17.3), when present, have a rim of

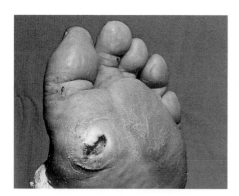

Figure 17.2 *Neuropathic ulcer with surrounding callus under the first metatarsophalangeal joint.*

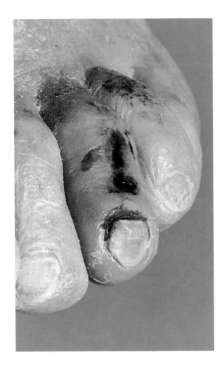

Figure 17.3 *Ischaemic ulcer on the dorsal surface of the third toe.*

erythema, which often turns black, and there is no build up of callus. In the ischaemic foot, tissue is devitalized and is particularly prone to rapid spread of infection. The sites most commonly affected are the medial surface of the head of the first metatarsal, the lateral surface of the head of the fifth metatarsal, other metatarsal heads and the heel. Gangrenous change is indicated by blackening of the toes or foot.

Assessment of the diabetic foot

The most important predictors of foot ulcers are:

- foot deformity (Table 17.1)
- neuropathy – identified by the inability to perceive a 10-g monofilament rod (Figure 17.4; Table 17.2) or light touch
- severe PVD.

These factors are most easily predicted through history and clinical examination. A protocol is suggested in Tables 17.2 and 17.3.

Table 17.1 Types of foot deformity and prevalence found in a community survey of diabetic patients (n = 635) aged 65 years and over[1]

Type of deformity	Definition*	Prevalence (%) Men	Women
Hallux valgus	Lateral deviation of the great toe at the MP joint	15.3	36.0
Claw toes	Fixed flexion deformity of proximal IP joint and distal IP joint Hyperextension of the MP joint	13.5	13.6
Pes cavus	High longitudinal arch with an angle between the forefoot and hindfoot approaching 90°	1.5	1.0
Hallux rigidus	Little movement on either flexion or extension of the MP joint		
Hammer toes	Fixed flexion deformity of proximal IP joint with hyperextension of distal IP and MP joints	17.7	15.6
Pes planus	Reduced longitudinal arch so that on standing, its medial border is in contact with the ground		
Total		48.6	66.2

*Definitions according to reference 1.

IP = interphalangeal; MP = metatarsophalangeal.

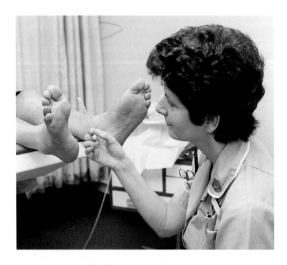

Figure 17.4 *Testing sensation with a monofilament.*

Management of diabetic foot disease

Patients who are considered at low risk of diabetic foot disease can be managed in primary care with regular chiropody and annual screening, but high-risk patients require referral (Tables 17.2 and 17.3).

Ulcer prevention programme

All diabetic patients should receive education about foot care (see panel). Those patients categorized as medium- or high-risk after assessment need further education. Ulcer prevention programmes can reduce the incidence of foot ulceration by 30%. The following features should be included in the programme:

- raising patient awareness of the risk of ulceration
- daily foot hygiene and self-examination
- fast and easy access to a diabetic foot clinic if problems are identified
- attention to footwear and provision of special insoles/footwear if required
- regular chiropody
- good glycaemic control

Looking after your feet
(for patients with diabetes)

1. Wash your feet every day and dry carefully between the toes. Inspect your feet daily using a mirror, if necessary, or ask someone else to check them for you. Your feet should not be 'soaked'. A simple aqueous cream (e.g. E45®) may be applied to the skin.

2. Cut toenails straight across after washing your feet. If your sight is not good, do not attempt it, but go to the chiropodist regularly. Explain that you have diabetes.

3. Do not walk around barefoot, particularly not on wooden floors.

4. Never use corn paint, plasters, salves or pads.

5. Make sure that your shoes fit well and have broad toes and low heels. Do not wear new shoes for more than half an hour at a time. Stockings and socks should be of natural fibre (cotton or wool), if possible, and washed in a fabric conditioner.

6. Avoid excessive heat or cold. To avoid being cold, wear thick socks (preferably clean every day) and long pants. Never put your feet closer to the fire than 4 feet (1.25 metres). Remove hot water bottles from the bed before getting in.

7. Report all sore places, blisters or discoloured areas to your doctor or practice nurse, however trivial they may seem to you.

8. Do not smoke.

By following these guidelines, the majority of serious foot troubles can be avoided.

- avoidance of smoking
- regular exercise for PVD.

Table 17.2 Annual neuropathy assessment of the feet

1 Test sensation: light touch or 10-g monofilament rod

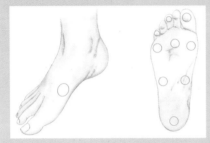 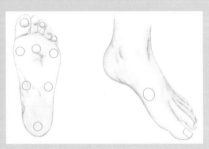

Number of points felt out of 10 _____   Number of points felt out of 10 _____

2 Does the patient have an ulcer?   Yes/No

3 Has the patient had a foot ulcer in the past?   Yes/No

4 Is the footwear suitable?   Yes/No

5 Any foot deformities in the past?   Right _____ Left _____

_____ _____

_____ _____

Risk category	**Management plan**
A No foot ulcer and no history of ulceration No foot deformity No neuropathy (≥ 80% test sites positive)	**A** Low risk Foot care advice Annual neuropathy assessment
B No foot ulcer, but past history of foot ulcer or Foot deformity or Evidence of neuropathy (< 80% test sites positive)	**B** Medium risk Examine feet each visit Refer to ulcer prevention programme and continuous re-education Regular chiropody
C Foot ulcer present with or without Foot deformity or Evidence of neuropathy (< 80% test sites positive)	**C** High risk Immediate urgent referral to diabetic foot clinic Long term: ulcer prevention programme and regular chiropody

The chiropodist, diabetes nurse specialist and practice nurse are ideal members of the team to direct an ulcer prevention programme.

The diabetologist or family practitioner should also review management of PVD, considering aspirin and anti-hyperlipidaemia treatment (see Chapter 15).

Management of established ulceration

All diabetic patients found to have a foot ulcer, breach of skin (e.g. blister), or area of suspected ischaemia or gangrene should be referred urgently to the diabetic foot clinic (or the diabetologist if there is no local established foot clinic). These patients need to be seen quickly (within a maximum of 1 week) as infection can spread rapidly and lead to avoidable amputation. The main features of treatment provided by a team approach include:

- clinical assessment of the foot using Doppler measurements and radiography as appropriate
- expert chiropody with callus removal and necrotic tissue debridement
- intensive antibiotic therapy
- establishment of excellent glycaemic control with frequent home monitoring
- assessment and provision of appropriate footwear
- appropriate referral to a vascular surgeon for angiography and revascularization
- appropriate definitive surgery if amputation is required.

The primary health care team, and particularly the district nurse, will be involved in this team approach. The specialist diabetic foot clinics have shown that it is possible to reduce amputation rates dramatically and to promote early healing of foot ulcers.

The importance of chiropody

The importance of expert chiropody cannot be overemphasized. The chiropodist must be state registered and adequately trained for the care of patients with diabetes. Broadly speaking, chiropodists may be divided into two groups: those working in the community and specialist chiropodists working at the diabetic foot clinic.

Table 17.3 Annual vascular assessment of the feet

1 Are foot pulses palpable?

	Right	Left
Dorsalis pedis	Yes/No	Yes/No
Posterior tibial	Yes/No	Yes/No

2 Doppler measurement of ankle brachial pressure index (ABPI) if foot pulses weak or absent:

$$ABPI^* = \frac{\text{ankle systolic pressure}^{**}}{\text{brachial systolic pressure}}$$

Right ABPI = _____   Left ABPI = _____

3 Any symptoms of intermittent claudication?

Right   Yes/No   Left   Yes/No

4 Does the patient have rest pain?

Right   Yes/No   Left   Yes/No

Risk category	**Management plan**
I Palpable foot pulses or ABPI > 0.9 No claudication or rest pain	**I** Low risk Annual vascular foot assessment
II ABPI between 0.5 and 0.9 No claudication or rest pain	**II** Medium risk Examine feet each visit Review smoking, lipids, drugs and aspirin treatment Ulcer prevention programme

III History of claudication
and ABPI < 0.9

III High risk
Refer to vascular surgeon
Review smoking, lipids, drugs
and aspirin treatment
Examine feet each visit
Ulcer prevention programme

IV Presence of ischaemic ulcer or
Rest pain or ABPI < 0.5

IV High risk
Immediate referral to diabetic foot
clinic for urgent review, including
assessment by vascular surgeon

*Falsely high ABPI may be due to vessel calcification caused by autonomic neuropathy.
**Highest systolic reading from dorsalis pedis or posterior tibial artery.

Mixed neuropathy and vascular risk categories

Neuropathy risk category B + Vascular risk category II or III: Refer to diabetic foot clinic

Specialist chiropodists are trained to undertake minor surgery and the expert care and management of diabetic foot disease. The chiropodist is an essential part of the team without whom the diabetic foot clinic could not function. The diabetic foot clinic chiropodist should be involved in:

- initial education
- initial assessment
- intensive investigation and treatment of those at risk of or with established foot disease
- footwear assessment and fitting
- follow-up and maintenance of high-risk patients.

Prevention of diabetic foot disease

In no part of the service is education of diabetic patients more important. Foot care education should form part of the initial education programme (see page 42) by diabetes specialist nurses and chiropodists. This should be followed by individual assessment by the chiropodist.

In primary care, regular screening for neuropathy, PVD, foot deformity and diabetic foot disease should be carried out annually. Regular chiropody within the community should be available and provided on a routine basis for those who require it. High-risk patients identified in primary care should be referred to the diabetic foot clinic.

Shared care summary

■ Diabetic foot disease is common and may lead to ulceration and amputation.

■ Foot deformity, neuropathy and/or PVD are risk factors for diabetic foot disease.

■ All diabetic patients should be educated about foot care and have their feet examined annually.

■ A careful history and examination of the feet can identify 'at risk' patients.

■ 'At risk' patients should attend an ulcer prevention programme run by the chiropodist, diabetes nurse specialist and/or practice nurse.

■ All diabetic patients with a foot ulcer, breach of the skin or suspicion of ischaemia should be referred urgently to the diabetic foot clinic.

■ Diabetic foot disease requires intensive management with expert chiropody, antibiotics, excellent glycaemic control, regular dressings and appropriate footwear. Dressings are commonly applied by the district nurse or practice nurse.

■ Patients with significant PVD require referral to a vascular surgeon for assessment, angiography and revascularization, if appropriate.

Reference

1 Walters DP, Gatling W, Hill RD, Mullee MA. The prevalence of foot deformity in diabetic subjects: a population study in an English community. *Practical Diabetes* 1993; **10:** 106–8.

Further reading

Boulton AJM, Connor H, Cavanagh PR, eds. *The foot in diabetes. 2nd edn.* Chichester: John Wiley & Sons, 1994.

Schaper NC, Bakker K, eds. *The diabetic foot. Proceedings of the Second International Symposium on the Diabetic Foot, Noordwijkerhout, The Netherlands, 10–12 May 1995. Diabet Med* 1996; **13** (Suppl 1): S1–64.

Chapter 18

Planning and auditing diabetes care

Some aspects of diabetes care planning, execution and audit are considered in this chapter. The responsibilities of both primary and secondary health care sectors, their coordination and integration are outlined along with, most importantly, the responsibilities of the patient. Whether diabetes care is successful can only be assessed by auditing the process and the outcome, preferably at district level. The development of a satisfactory auditing system is described and the importance of such a system for improvements in standards of care is discussed.

Organization of diabetes care

The total care of patients with diabetes involves a large number of people (both health care professionals and lay people) acting at different sites (Table 18.1). Responsibilities for care may be shared between:

■ the patient (or carer)
■ the primary health care team (PHCT)
■ the secondary health care team.

Patient co-operation booklets facilitate communication between all three groups (see pages 135–6). The most important person in the complete health care team is, however, the diabetic patient.

Patient responsibilities

Provided that the patient has reasonable intelligence, education and social background, his/her responsibilities might be expected to include:

Table 18.1 People involved in the total care of patients with diabetes

Patients' homes
- Patients
- Relatives and friends

Primary care and the community
- Family doctors
- Practice nurses
- Secretaries
- Receptionists and managers
- District nurses
- Community dietitian
- Community chiropodists
- Ophthalmic medical practitioners and ophthalmic opticians (optometrists)
- Community pharmacists
- Psychologists

Secondary health care
- Diabetologists and other specialists
- Diabetes specialist nurses, clinic nurses, midwives and ward nurses
- Dietitians
- Chiropodists
- Receptionists, secretaries, clerks (appointments and medical records)
- Pharmacists
- Laboratory staff
- Radiography department staff
- Telephonists
- Administrators

- management of his/her own diabetic status (with the help of others)
- acquisition of necessary knowledge and skills
- active pursuit of follow-up for glycaemic control review and for prevention, screening and treatment of complications.

Patients need constant support from relatives, friends and health care personnel. Those who are not fortunate enough to be able to acquire the necessary skills and discipline require extra help and care.

PHCT responsibilities

The PHCT have wide-ranging responsibilities to the diabetic patient (Table 18.2), covering not only clinical aspects (diagnosis, monitoring, referral, and early detection of complications) but also education and reassurance.

Organization of diabetes care within primary care: diabetes care needs to be structured, but there are several different ways of achieving an efficient system. In some practices, one family practitioner may opt to become the 'diabetes expert', working closely with a practice nurse, who also develops appropriate skills. In other practices, all family practitioners may undertake diabetes care for their patients. Some practices set up dedicated miniclinics, while others undertake diabetes care in normal surgery hours but follow a protocol to ensure good care.

In the UK, the Department of Health[1] has published guidelines for organizing diabetes care in general practice. In summary, the practice should:

- keep an up-to-date register of all patients with diabetes
- ensure systematic call and recall of these patients to the practice or see that it is undertaken at the hospital
- provide appropriate education and advice for newly diagnosed diabetic patients either in the practice or by referral to the hospital
- ensure that all diabetic patients receive continuing education
- ensure that at initial diagnosis and at least annually, a full review is carried out

Table 18.2 Responsibilities of the PHCT towards the diabetic patient

■ To maintain a high index of suspicion and detect diabetes at an early stage

■ To confirm the diagnosis of diabetes mellitus according to WHO criteria

■ To initiate first aid treatment and begin the educational process (family doctor to be sympathetic and reassuring)

■ To ensure patients receive proper education, either at the hospital or in primary care

■ To monitor and revise treatment in order to achieve satisfactory standards of glycaemic control

■ To provide routine follow-up to assess the standard of glycaemic control (minimum 6-monthly intervals) and to detect at an early stage any long-term complications or risk factors for complications (annual review)

■ To refer patients for review when problems either occur or are foreseen

■ To provide an efficient appointment and recall system that will identify patients who fail to attend

■ To provide a domiciliary service for the elderly

■ To organize practice and community nurses to provide domiciliary help

■ To liaise fully with the secondary health care team

■ agree with each patient an individual management plan, including the choice of long-term follow-up, which should be recorded on the register

■ refer patients to secondary care when appropriate and also to relevant support agencies

■ work together with other professionals, such as dietitians and chiropodists, to ensure that the practice team is appropriately trained in the management of diabetes

■ maintain an adequate record of the process of care and its outcomes, including information from other people involved in patient care

■ audit the care of patients with diabetes against the above criteria.

Secondary health care responsibilities

The hospital based service should provide the following[2]:

■ diabetes education facilities

■ initial review and assessment

■ open access laboratory services

■ special follow-up clinics for problems and complications (Table 18.3)

■ assessment of new problems

■ specialist chiropody service (linked to diabetic foot clinic)

■ specialist dietetic service (linked to education service)

■ facilities for monitoring and audit, preferably computer based, for the whole district.

Secondary health care responsibilities are probably best discharged from a diabetes centre (Figure 18.1).

Table 18.3 Special follow-up clinics to be organized by the secondary health care team to cope with specific problems

■ Diabetic eye disease

■ Diabetic renal disease

■ Diabetic foot disease

■ Routine diabetic follow-up clinic for patients with problems of glycaemic control or other problems not covered at specific clinics

■ Joint diabetic/obstetric clinic

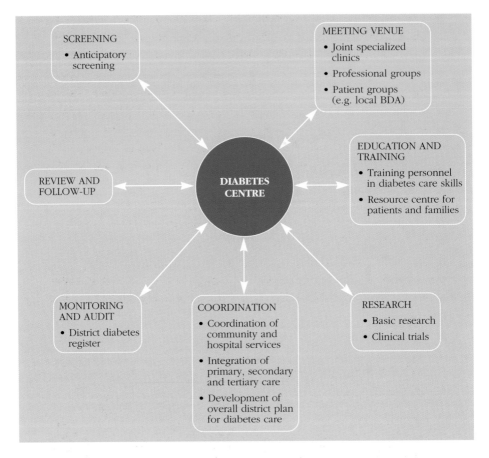

SCREENING
• Anticipatory screening

MEETING VENUE
• Joint specialized clinics
• Professional groups
• Patient groups (e.g. local BDA)

DIABETES CENTRE

EDUCATION AND TRAINING
• Training personnel in diabetes care skills
• Resource centre for patients and families

REVIEW AND FOLLOW-UP

MONITORING AND AUDIT
• District diabetes register

COORDINATION
• Coordination of community and hospital services
• Integration of primary, secondary and tertiary care
• Development of overall district plan for diabetes care

RESEARCH
• Basic research
• Clinical trials

Figure 18.1 *Functions of a district diabetes centre*[2].

Coordination and integration

Coordination and integration are two essential prerequisites of effective diabetes care, though they may be difficult to achieve.

Although the diabetes specialist is naturally the leader in a particular district, his/her role is impossible without the full support and encouragement of PHCTs. The diabetologist should assume responsibility for the organization and integration of the service as a whole and take a leading role in the local services diabetes advisory group. This role should include the collection of demographic data in the district served by the hospital in order to make future projections and assess future needs. Assessment of the current status of the service and its deficiencies is an essential prerequisite for a plan of action to remedy faults.

In addition to provision of the patient-centred programme in the diabetes centre, the diabetologist should also organize educational facilities and a forum for discussion for the PHCTs. Joint meetings between the PHCTs and the Diabetes Centre Team (Figure 18.2) should be arranged on a regular basis. At these meetings, the following topics are advisable points for discussion:

- service problems and their potential solutions
- recent research advances and clinical update
- monitoring and audit
- appreciation of each others' problems.

Similar meetings should be held with optometrists and ophthalmic medical practitioners if they are involved in screening for diabetic eye disease.

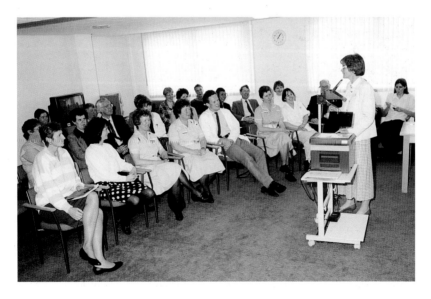

Figure 18.2 *A joint meeting of diabetes teams from both primary and secondary care.*

Monitoring the St Vincent Declaration targets[3] (see page 12) entails assessment of diabetes mortality and morbidity among the local population. The development of a district diabetes register is very important and must naturally involve cooperation between primary and secondary care. Each practice register needs to be maintained to a high degree of accuracy with regular updating. In turn, this needs to be linked to the district diabetes register to ensure two-way updating.

Auditing diabetes care

It has been said that research is concerned with discovering the right thing to do, while audit is concerned with ensuring that it is rightly done[4]. It is important not to confuse the two. Audit should in fact be carried out for one reason only, namely to improve the standard of patient care.

Audit definitions

The definitions given below may help to avoid confusion.

Audit is an objective and systematic method of evaluating the quality of health care, with the aim of identifying and implementing opportunities for improvement in the professional performance of those auditing their work.

Medical audit activities are concerned with the performance of doctors.

Clinical audit is the audit of any aspect of clinical care provided by members of the health care team. Diabetes care is a team activity and requires clinical rather than medical audit.

Audit of structure (input) is a measure of the resources used in diabetes care. It is done in order to compare the resources

234

available in one practice with those in another, in the local diabetes service and with the criteria defined nationally, for example, by the British Diabetic Association (BDA). Such comparisons may be useful for the negotiation of improvements in the resources for diabetes care.

Process audit is a measurement of what is actually done during the process of care. The BDA has suggested that all diabetic patients should have the following tests or examinations performed annually:

■ assessment of glycaemic control (e.g. determination of HbA_{1C})
■ measurement of blood pressure
■ examination of the eyes
■ examination of the feet
■ measurement of renal function (e.g. serum creatinine)
■ test for proteinuria
■ assessment of lipid status (e.g. serum cholesterol)

The date on which each of these processes is carried out becomes the audit indicator (see below) for that process.

Outcome audit is a measure of what is actually achieved. Mortality and morbidity are probably the most valid long-term outcome measures. For short-term outcome assessment, surrogate indicators known to influence both morbidity and mortality may be used (e.g. HbA_{1C}, urinary albumin or microalbuminuria, serum cholesterol, blood pressure, body mass index).

Audit indicators are specifically defined measurements used in audit, though in general practice, the term 'criterion' is often used instead of 'audit indicator'[5]. For diabetes care in the UK, these have been agreed nationally[6].

Definition of standard

In an ideal world, all patients would receive ideal care and a perfect outcome would be achieved (e.g. 100% of patients would have their eyes examined annually and all cases of blindness would be prevented). In the real world, this is not possible. Although 100% must be the ultimate goal, a realistic standard should be set. Attempts should then be made to improve on the standards set and the audit repeated to measure any improvement.

Data collection

Manual data collection by scrutiny of notes is laborious, time consuming and expensive. As audit is an ongoing process and needs repeating at intervals, an integrated audit system is essential and a computerized database is the best option.

One suitable software program for audit analysis is DIALOG[7,8], which is not a clinical information system, but may be used merely for the manipulation of data and the provision of a valid analysis. It is most useful at district, regional or national levels, when sufficient data can be obtained to allow valid statistical comparisons.

The audit cycle

The processes of observing clinical practice, measuring audit indicators and assessing the results form but the first part of the audit cycle. If the audit indicates that there is room for improvement in care, then clinical practice must be changed. The effects of any changes are then assessed over a period of time by measurement of audit indicators. This process forms a cycle of events (the audit cycle) aimed at the gradual improvement of care (Table 18.4).

Audit interpretation

Great care must be taken in the interpretation of results of an audit, particularly with respect to comparisons between practices. The following pitfalls should be avoided.

■ The audit indicators must be measured identically.

■ The audit periods must be similar.

Table 18.4 Stages in performing an audit

1 Define precisely the purpose of the audit and set standards

2 Identify the nature of the audit:
- structure
- process
- outcome

3 Select and define the audit indicators

4 Define how data are to be:
- collected
- stored
- analysed
- assessed

5 Set the audit time period

6 Assess the cost in terms of time, manpower and finance. Will your budget stand it?

7 Commence the audit

8 Analyse the results

9 Present the results to the team for discussion

10 Decide on any necessary changes to clinical practice

11 Implement the changes

12 Repeat the audit

- The audit populations must be similar with respect to age, sex, ethnic structure, proportions with insulin dependent and non-insulin dependent diabetes, and other factors.

- Sufficient numbers of patients must be included for statistically significant results to be obtained.

- The development and constant maintenance of a District Diabetes Register is an essential component of successful district audit.

Shared care summary

■ Responsibility for lifelong care of a patient with diabetes must be shared between the PHCT, the hospital diabetes team and the patient (or carer).

■ The PHCT have wide-ranging responsibilities, including diagnosis, follow-up, education and reassurance.

■ Responsibilities of the hospital-based team include education (of both patients and professionals), screening, follow-up and specialist diabetes management.

■ Organization and integration of care should be led by the district diabetes specialist, who should arrange regular joint meetings between the PHCTs and the hospital based team.

■ The PHCT must be responsible for the establishment and updating of a practice diabetes register, while the district register is the responsibility of the hospital based team. Computerized interlinking of the two registers allows efficient updating.

■ Cooperation between primary and secondary care is imperative so that efficient district based diabetes audit is possible.

■ The audit cycle consists of setting standards, carrying out an audit, assessing results, implementing necessary changes to practice, resetting standards and repeating the audit.

■ The primary aim of diabetes audit is to improve the quality of care for patients with diabetes.

References

1 NHS Management Executive. *General practice contract and health promotion package: guidance and implementation, 1993.*

2 Clinical Standards Advisory Group. *Standards of clinical care for people with diabetes.* London: HMSO, 1994.

3 Piwernetz K, Home PD, Snorgaard O, Antsiferov M, Staehr-Johansen K, Krans M for the DIABCARE Monitoring Group of the St Vincent Declaration Steering Committee. Monitoring the targets of the St Vincent Declaration and the implementation of quality management in diabetes care: the DIABCARE initiative. *Diabet Med* 1993; **10:** 371–7.

4 Smith R. Audit and research. *BMJ* 1992; **305:** 905–6.

5 Royal College of General Practitioners. *Quality and audit in general practice; meanings and definitions.* London: Royal College of General Practitioners, 1990.

6 Wilson AE, Home PD, for the Diabetes Audit Working Group of the Research Unit of the Royal College of Physicians and the British Diabetic Association. A dataset to allow exchange of information for monitoring continuing diabetes care. *Diabet Med* 1993; **10:** 378–90.

7 Vaughan NJA, Shaw M, Boer F, Billett D, Martin C. Creation of a district diabetes register using the DIALOG system. *Diabet Med* 1996; **13:** 175–81.

8 Vaughan NJA, Hopkinson N, Christy VA. DIALOG: coordination of the annual review process through a district diabetes register linked to the FHSA database. *Diabet Med* 1996; **13:** 182–8.

Further reading

Alexander W, Bradshaw C, Gadsby R *et al.* for the British Diabetic Association. An approach to manageable datasets in diabetes care. *Diabet Med* 1994; **11:** 806–10.

British Diabetic Association, Diabetes Services Advisory Committee. *Recommendations for the management of diabetes in primary care.* London: British Diabetic Association, 1993.

Vaughan NJA, for the Audit Working Group of the Research Unit of the Royal College of Physicians and British Diabetic Association, and the Centre for Health Services Research, University of Newcastle upon Tyne. Measuring the outcomes of diabetes care. *Diabet Med* 1994; **11:** 418–23.

Chapter 19

Future developments in diabetes care

Striking advances have been made in the care of diabetic patients during the last 30 years, and the future is even more exciting. The realization that insulin dependent diabetes mellitus (IDDM) is an autoimmune disease with a long period of development before becoming clinically significant has opened up a host of possibilities for prevention and treatment.

The incidence and prevalence of diabetes is increasing across the world. Although this applies to both types of diabetes, in terms of numbers of people affected, the increase in non-insulin dependent diabetes (NIDDM) is creating a greater impact. Better understanding of the cause of NIDDM and the risk factors important to its development could lead to major population strategies for its prevention.

IDDM

IDDM used to be thought to have a fairly acute onset, but it has emerged that patients may be under immune attack for a decade or more before signs or symptoms appear. The clinical onset of the disease is often precipitated by the added stress of trauma or infection. The occurrence of a detectable sub-clinical phase of the disease (Figure 19.1) may offer a strategy for screening with a view to its prevention. Various serum markers, such as islet cell antibodies (ICA), insulin auto-antibodies and anti-64kDa antibodies, are present before the overt onset of IDDM. Screening for such markers is one way of identifying at-risk people.

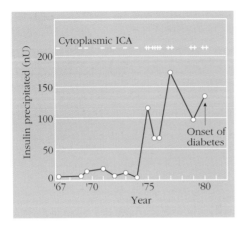

Figure 19.1 *Appearance of antibody markers 5 years before the onset of IDDM in a monozygotic twin of a diabetic patient. Reproduced with permission from Soeldner JS et al., 1985[1].*

Screening families with a history of IDDM would identify only a limited number of at-risk people as only 10% of those developing IDDM have a family history of the disease. Population screening is required, but would be expensive. The age at which screening should be undertaken also needs to be established. Recent work has identified the presence of autoantibodies even at birth[2].

Prevention of IDDM development

Primary prevention of IDDM would involve elimination of the environmental factors involved in initiation of the autoimmune process, while secondary prevention would involve aborting the autoimmune response that is responsible for islet cell destruction. One primary preventive measure that has been undertaken on a national scale is the avoidance of milk protein in Finland, where it has been documented that diabetic children show a high prevalence of anti-bovine albumin antibodies – bovine albumin being a protein normally present in cows' milk. The idea is to evaluate the effect of milk protein avoidance on IDDM incidence.

For months or years before IDDM development, metabolic and immunological changes are apparent, and their detection gives a prior warning period during which it may be possible to engage secondary prevention of the progression to frank diabetes. Several approaches focusing on the autoimmune nature of the disease are currently under investigation.

Immunosuppressive therapy: current immunosuppressive drugs (e.g. azathioprine, cyclosporin) have already been tried with some success in patients with recently diagnosed IDDM. Side-effects of immunosuppressive drugs, such as nephrotoxicity and increased risk of infection, have limited their use, which is potentially more harmful than insulin treatment. Moreover, they appear only to delay the inevitable return of IDDM rather than to prevent it completely.

Antioxidants: as free radicals, particularly nitric oxide, are in some way involved in islet cell destruction by activated T cells, antioxidants have been proposed as protective factors for people in the prediabetic state. Nicotinamide (vitamin B_3), desferrioxamine and probucol are antioxidants that have all proved effective in protecting islet cells from destruction in animal studies or cell culture experiments.

Nicotinamide may also help to prevent IDDM development by increasing insulin synthesis and stimulating regeneration of pancreatic β-cells. Several trials are investigating either the protective effect of nicotinamide in high-risk children (e.g. the German Nicotinamide Intervention Study or DENIS) or at various ages (e.g. the large double-blind European Nicotinamide Diabetes Intervention Trial or ENDIT).

Insulin therapy: insulin treatment in animals has been found to delay the development of diabetes, a possible explanation being reduced susceptibility of β-cells to immune attack when they are resting rather than secreting insulin. Accordingly, trials involving treatment with insulin before diabetes develops are underway in the USA. High-risk individuals (i.e. those with a 50% chance of developing diabetes within 5 years) are being recruited.

Treatment of IDDM

The ideal treatment for IDDM remains elusive. Pancreatic transplantation is a well established technique but graft survival is less than optimal: 75% at 1 year and 65% at 5 years. The requirement for immunosuppressive therapy and the significant risk of graft failure prohibit its general recommendation, except for patients undergoing renal transplantation. The developing field of islet cell transplantation has greater promise. The technique involves the injection of islet cells into the portal vein with subsequent seeding in the liver. At present, patients require immunosuppressive therapy to prevent rejection and delay autoimmune damage to the seeded islet cells. The development of a membrane to encapsulate the islet cells and protect them from immune attack, while allowing glucose sensing and insulin secretion, is in progress.

Another achievable goal is the development of an implantable artificial pancreas, which current progress in microelectronics has rendered potentially successful. The ability to monitor blood glucose continuously and non-invasively has so far been the stumbling block, though the development of implantable glucose sensors is accelerating in the USA with a view to widespread patient use by the end of the decade. Addition of a hypoglycaemia alarm and linkage to an implantable, refillable insulin pump, which is already available, to form a closed loop insulin delivery system (i.e. an artificial pancreas) finally seems possible.

New insulin preparations are being investigated. Research is focusing on the construction of insulin analogues, perhaps with only one or two amino acids changed, that exist preferentially as dimers or monomers. Insulin normally aggregates into hexamers; the dimeric form is absorbed faster and the monomeric form fastest of all. Moreover, it is the monomeric form that binds to insulin receptors. As the absorption of these analogues is faster and their duration of action shorter (Figure 19.2), they would be particularly useful for multiple injection therapy (MIT; see page 98). One such analogue, insulin lispro, has been released for clinical use in the UK in 1996. Clinical trials have so far shown it to be as effective as

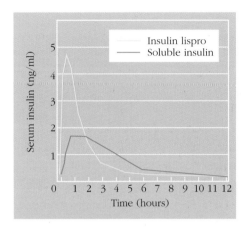

Figure 19.2 *Rapid absorption of insulin lispro in comparison with soluble insulin resulting in more rapid attainment of peak serum insulin levels*[3].

soluble insulin with one study reporting fewer hypoglycaemic episodes when insulin lispro was used in an MIT regimen[3]. Its place in treating patients with IDDM should become clearer with more extensive use.

NIDDM

NIDDM is the end stage of a process that evolves over many years. Indeed, patients presenting with complications are believed to have had the disease possibly for 7 years or more (Figure 19.3)[4]. Longitudinal studies have explored predictors of impaired glucose tolerance (IGT) and NIDDM, and also protective influences (Table 19.1).

Early detection and treatment of NIDDM should reduce the rate at which complications develop. Early detection might be achieved by identifying high-risk individuals by selection from a local or regional computerized database and then undertaking screening. Primary care is particularly well placed to take on this role, as patients with particular characteristics may be easily identified from the practice register. Early treatment may be possible in patients with IGT; a new class of drug, thiazolidinedione (e.g. troglitazone), which acts by reducing insulin resistance, has been shown in clinical trials to reduce plasma glucose and insulin levels (Figure 19.4). Interestingly, there was a significant reduction in blood pressure during treatment. Other

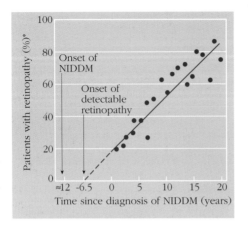

Figure 19.3 *Prevalence of retinopathy in people with NIDDM in the USA relative to the time of diagnosis of diabetes. Adapted from Harris MI et al., 1992[4].*

Table 19.1 Environmental factors and patient characteristics influencing the development of IGT and NIDDM

Increased risk
- Intra-uterine growth retardation
  Low birth weight
  Low weight at 1 year
- High body mass index (BMI)
  Increased central obesity
- Cigarette smoking
- Hypertension
- Ischaemic heart disease

Reduced risk
- High birthweight
  High weight at 1 year
- Low BMI
  Lean physique
- Greater physical activity
- Moderate alcohol intake

drugs in development (Table 19.2) will also open up new possibilities for the treatment of IGT and NIDDM.

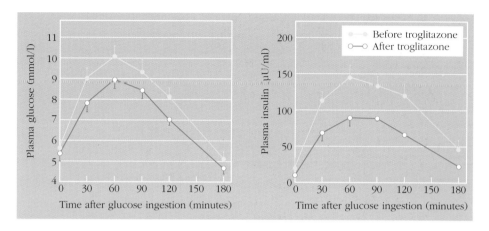

Figure 19.4 *Oral glucose tolerance tests in obese non-diabetic people (50% of whom had IGT) before and after treatment for 12 weeks with troglitazone. Results are mean ± SEM. Adapted from Nolan JJ et al., 1994[5].*

Table 19.2 Future drugs for treatment of NIDDM

- Insulin secretagogues, which act like sulphonylureas
- Agents, such as thiazolidinediones (e.g. ciglitazone, troglitazone), that reduce insulin resistance
- Inhibitors of hepatic gluconeogenesis that reduce glucose output from the liver
- Agents that stimulate weight loss (e.g. appetite suppressants, thermogenic agents)
- Lipid lowering drugs
- Inhibitors of digestive enzymes, such as α-glucosidase, amylase, lipases*

*Also for IDDM treatment.

In the long term, prevention of NIDDM must be the ultimate goal. This involves changes in both individual and population behaviour, with obesity reduction and increased physical activity. In underdeveloped areas, education and improvement in the nutritional status of pregnant women and children during their early growth years may be influential in reducing the risk of future NIDDM. Once again, the primary care health team has a crucial part to play in this area.

Shared care in diabetes

It is well recognized in medicine that although research may provide knowledge on superior management of a disease, there is often too long a gap between publication of research results and their incorporation into routine practice. The development of effective shared care may help to minimize this gap as members of different health care sectors work together as a team and promote mutual education. The central role of patients themselves should not be overlooked. Their experience of the disease should be recognized; it also has a role in the education of health care professionals.

Shared care summary

■ Research is currently opening up new possibilities for prevention and treatment of diabetes.

■ The autoimmune nature of IDDM and its prolonged subclinical phase offer scope for screening and prevention.

■ Trials to prevent IDDM are underway with antioxidants (e.g. nicotinamide) or insulin therapy.

■ Pancreatic transplantation is limited by poor graft survival and the need for immunosuppressive therapy; encapsulated β-cells may prove the transplant success of the future.

■ An implantable artificial pancreas, which is currently under development, may be fully functional within 5–10 years.

■ Insulin analogues, with faster absorption and action, are already being developed and marketed.

■ Early detection and treatment of NIDDM should reduce the incidence of complications.

■ Various approaches to the treatment of NIDDM offer sound prospects for the future.

■ Primary care has a vital role to play in the prevention of diabetes by promotion of healthy behavioural change, education and early diagnosis of IGT and NIDDM.

■ Improved patient management involving shared care will contribute to future advances.

References

1 Soeldner JS, Tuttleman M, Srikanta S, Ganda OP, Eisenbarth GS. Insulin-dependent diabetes mellitus and autoimmunity: islet-cell autoantibodies, insulin autoantibodies, and beta-cell failure. *N Engl J Med* 1985; **313:** 893–4.

2 Millward BA, Fewstor D, Wilkin TJ. Insulin binding in cord blood appears to be true IAA: the Earlybird Study. *Diabet Med* 1996; **13** (Suppl 3): S44.

3 Garg SK, Carmain JA, Braddy KC *et al.* Pre-meal insulin analogue insulin lispro vs Humulin® R insulin treatment in young subjects with Type 1 diabetes. *Diabet Med* 1996; **13:** 47–52.

4 Harris MI, Klein RE, Welborn TA, Knuiman MW. Onset of NIDDM occurs at least 4–7 years before clinical diagnosis. *Diabetes Care* 1992; **15:** 815–19.

5 Nolan JJ, Ludvik B, Beerdsen P, Joyce M, Olefsky J. Improvement in glucose tolerance and insulin resistance in obese subjects treated with troglitazone. *N Engl J Med* 1994; **331:** 1188–93.

6 Lau *et al.* Cumulative meta-analysis of therapeutic trials for myocardial infarction *New Engl J Med* 1992; **327(4):** 348.

Further reading

Eastman RC, Seaton T. Pharmacological approaches to non-insulin-dependent diabetes: future directions. In: Leslie RGD, Robbins DC, eds. *Diabetes: clinical science in practice*. Cambridge: Cambridge University Press, 1995: 353–9.

Pozzilli P. Strategies for the prevention of insulin-dependent diabetes. In: Leslie RGD, Robbins DC, eds. *Diabetes: clinical science in practice*. Cambridge: Cambridge University Press, 1995: 392–404.

Chapter 20

Shared care in practice: case studies

Case 1: Hypoglycaemia with a sulphonylurea

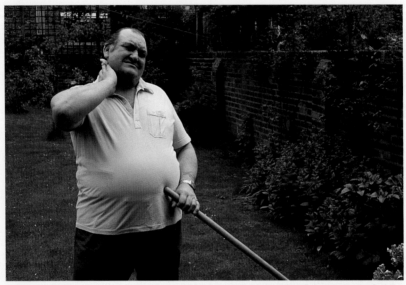

Reproduced with permission from Collections/Anthea Sieveking

A 48-year-old man presented with a 6-week history of thirst and fatigue. Although overweight (92 kg; height 168 cm; BMI 32.6 kg/m²), he had lost 5 kg over the previous few weeks.

Family practitioner. This patient had no significant past medical history. A urine sample showed 2% glycosuria and no ketones. I arranged for a laboratory plasma glucose test 2 hours after breakfast the following day.

The plasma glucose result confirmed the diagnosis of diabetes and indeed was so high (27.5 mmol/l) that I prescribed glibenclamide, 5 mg/day, to start immediately. He was advised to follow a low-sugar diet and given an appointment with the dietitian the following week.

Dietitian. This patient was given a weight reducing diet of about 2200 kcal/day and low in fat. He agreed to drink only sugar-free drinks, despite his dislike of them.

Family practitioner. At the follow-up consultation 1 month later, the patient reported mid-morning symptoms of tiredness, sweating and confusion, which were relieved by eating biscuits. He had gained over 1 kg in weight. The regular hypoglycaemic episodes prompted me to discontinue the glibenclamide. When reviewed 3 months later, the patient's urine tests were consistently negative and his weight was stable. The laboratory fasting glucose (5.8 mmol/l) and HbA_{1c} (5.7%; normal range 4.1–6.5%) confirmed good glycaemic control. As his blood glucose was so high at presentation, I was surprised that this patient's diabetes could possibly be controlled by diet alone.

Diabetologist. An initially high blood glucose does not always predict the need for oral hypoglycaemic agents (OHAs). It is wise to take a brief dietary history in such circumstances. The response to the thirst induced by the diabetes is often to drink large quantities of sugary drinks, and this patient confesses to a dislike of sugar-free drinks. Cutting down the simple sugar intake and adhering to a weight reducing diet often results in good control, partly due to a changed diet and partly due to increased insulin sensitivity.

In this patient the sulphonylurea had its two common side-effects: weight gain and hypoglycaemia. It is advisable to warn the patient of possible hypoglycaemia when introducing a sulphonylurea.

A sound approach for a patient with very high blood glucose is to start with diet alone and reassess after a short interval. Only if heavy glycosuria and symptoms of polyuria and thirst persist should an OHA be prescribed. For an obese patient, metformin is first-line therapy and will not cause hypoglycaemia. A sulphonylurea is appropriate for a non-obese patient.

Case 2: Insulin dependence in the older patient

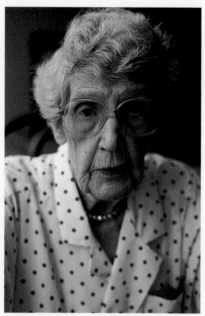

Reproduced with permission from Robert Hardy Picture Library

A 75-year-old woman presented to her family doctor shortly after her husband's death complaining of thirst, polyuria and rapid weight loss (6 kg in 2 months).

Family practitioner. This patient had been in fairly good health apart from hypothyroidism, which had been treated for 20 years. Her body weight was 54 kg (body mass index, 23.5 kg/m²) and her urine showed 2% glycosuria and no ketones. A 2-hour postprandial plasma glucose was 15.5 mmol/l, confirming diabetes. She was advised to follow a low-sugar diet and referred to the local diabetes education programme. An early review was arranged in view of her recent bereavement and her distress at the diabetes diagnosis.

At a follow-up review 1 week later, neither her symptoms nor her glycosuria had abated. Her urine still showed no ketones but her weight had dropped a further 1 kg. She had also developed vaginal candidiasis. She was prescribed:

- treatment for candidiasis
- gliclazide, 80 mg daily.

After only marginal improvement over the following week, the gliclazide was increased stepwise to the maximum of 160 mg twice daily and arrangements were made for laboratory blood tests and attendance at the local diabetic clinic. I was confident that this patient's compliance with both tablets and diet were excellent, but she failed to respond to the sulphonylurea.

Treatment	Urinary glucose	Plasma glucose (mmol/l)	HbA$_{1C}$(%)*
At presentation	2%	15.5 (2-hour post-meal)	
Diet alone (1 week)	2%	—	—
Gliclazide, 80 mg/day	2%	—	—
Gliclazide, 80 mg b.d.	1–2%	—	—
Gliclazide, 160 mg b.d.	1–2%	11.0 (fasting)	12.5

*Normal range = 4.1–6.5%

Diabetologist. Despite maximizing the dose of sulphonylurea, it failed to work for this patient. It would be inappropriate to add metformin as she is not overweight. Insulin treatment is clearly required to control this woman's diabetes.

Twice-daily premixed insulins (e.g. Mixtard 30 or Humulin M3) in a pen device for ease of administration would appear to be the best approach for a patient of this age and lifestyle. The diabetes nurse specialist can supervise the changeover to insulin treatment and involve the district nurse, who could also undertake some blood glucose monitoring if the patient did not feel capable of taking this on. A further review by the dietitian would be advisable with the emphasis on between-meal snacks and avoidance of hypoglycaemia.

With hindsight, the outcome was predictable. The patient already has one autoimmune disorder – hypothyroidism, probably due to Hashimoto's thyroiditis. Her diabetes is probably autoimmune, that is, true insulin dependent diabetes mellitus (IDDM) as well. Earlier diagnosis in primary care and the insidious onset of IDDM (see page 241) may explain why so many more patients now present with IDDM without urinary ketones or ketoacidosis.

Case 3: 'Mild diabetes'

A 64-year-old man visited his optician for new glasses as his sight had been deteriorating. The optometrist carried out a full examination and advised a visit to the family practitioner as there was "evidence of diabetes affecting the back of his eyes." Apparently 5 years previously, he had been told that he had diabetes but that it was only mild. Although he had followed his diet at first, he had forgotten about it over the years.

Family practitioner. This patient moved into the area 3 years ago. He had slipped through the system as his name was not included in the practice diabetes register. The optometrist reported distant visual acuity of 6/12 right eye and 6/36 left eye, plus a bilateral exudative maculopathy. A full review was undertaken plus referral to an ophthalmologist.

The patient's diabetes was poorly controlled. He was overweight (body mass index, 32 kg/m^2) and smoked 20 cigarettes/day. His blood pressure (BP) was raised and he complained of claudication in his left leg at 100 yards. Peripheral pulses were absent in the left leg and there was evidence of neuropathy (viz. reduced light touch and vibration sense in both feet and absent ankle reflexes).

Results

	Urinary glucose	Urinary albumin	Plasma glucose (mmol/l)	HbA$_{1c}$(%)*	Serum creatinine (μmol/l)	BP
At first review	2%	0	12.5 (random)	—	—	180/105
Diet (1 month)	Negative	0	6.5 (fasting)	7.8	96	165/95– 180/100**
Diet (4 months) + amlodipine, 10 mg/day	Negative	0	6.2 (fasting)	6.4	—	144/85– 150/90**

*Normal range = 4.1–6.5%. **Measured by the practice nurse.

After a long discussion, in which the patient was advised to return to following his diet and to stop smoking, visits to both the dietitian and the practice nurse were arranged.

After 1 month, he was commenced on amlodipine, 5 mg/day, as BP results were consistently high. Glycaemic control was improving with diet alone, but the fasting lipid profile demonstrated a mixed hyperlipidaemia.

Fasting lipid profiles

	TC (mmol/l)	HDL (mmol/l)	TC:HDL*	Triglyceride (mmol/l)
Diet (1 month)	6.9	0.8	8.6	3.6
Diet (4 months)	7.2	0.9	8.0	3.0
Diet + fenofibrate (1 year)	6.0	1.1	5.5	1.9

HDL = high density lipoprotein cholesterol; TC = total cholesterol. *Normal TC:HDL ratio < 5.

Claudication in the left leg was a continuing problem, so the patient was commenced on aspirin, 75 mg/day, and referred to the vascular surgeon. Regular chiropody and foot care education were arranged in view of the combination of neuropathy and peripheral vascular disease.

Some 3 months later, when the hyperlipidaemia persisted, the patient was commenced on fenofibrate, 300 mg/day. Diabetes and hypertension both remained well controlled.

The next annual review was disappointing; despite laser photocoagulation, visual acuity had deteriorated to 6/18 right eye and 6/60 left eye. He had a myocardial infarction and planned vascular surgery on his left leg was postponed. He was retired from work on medical grounds and has become very depressed.

Diabetologist. This case highlights the myth of 'mild diabetes' and how patients can be misled regarding the seriousness of the situation. After a long period of hyperglycaemia due to poor diet, this patient developed complications. By the time he presented with complications, much damage had already occurred and treatment had only a limited effect.

It is important to educate all diabetic patients about the need for good glycaemic control, regular follow-up and screening for complications. Unfortunately, many patients with non-insulin dependent diabetes mellitus (NIDDM) do not receive the necessary information and education.

Case 4: Poor control delays healing

A woman who had had non-insulin dependent diabetes mellitus (NIDDM) controlled by diet alone for 5 years had a scarring rash on her legs. A minor injury to her shin broke the skin and when it did not heal over 2 weeks, she presented to the practice nurse for treatment.

Practice nurse. The scarring rash was due to necrobiosis lipoidica diabeticorum, which resulted in thin skin on the shin area and ulceration after injury. The ulcerated area was swabbed and dressed and, after discussion with the family practitioner, she was prescribed a course of flucloxacillin. *Staphylococcus aureus* was cultured from the swab and was sensitive to flucloxacillin. Over the following 4 weeks, the ulcer did not heal, despite regular dressing, so the patient was referred to the local diabetes centre.

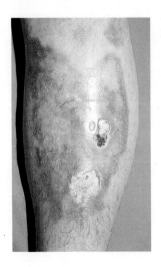

Ulcerated necrobiosis lipoidica diabeticorum.

Diabetologist. Necrobiosis lipoidica diabeticorùm is a skin problem associated with diabetes. Although some dermatologists advise injection of steroids into the edges of the lesions, I have no experience of this proving successful.

This patient had an infected ulcerated area with necrotic slough at its base. After swabbing, the ulcer was debrided and a desloughing dressing applied. Combined flucloxacillin and ampicillin (co-fluampicil), 2 tablets q.d.s., was prescribed pending the result of the swab culture. Ulcer healing was delayed by a combination of infection and poorly controlled diabetes. The patient's own urine tests showed 1–2% glycosuria and laboratory tests confirmed poor control (random plasma glucose, 12.5 mmol/l; HbA_{1C}, 9.5%, normal range 4.1–6.5%). Gliclazide, 40 mg/day, was commenced and the patient was reviewed by the dietitian.

At a follow-up consultation 1 week later, the urine test results had improved to ¼–½% glycosuria. Control was clearly not optimal, so the gliclazide dose was increased to 80 mg/day. Within 1 week, urine tests became negative without any symptoms of hypoglycaemia. As the wound swab culture showed a mixed growth, including *S. aureus*, the co-fluampicil was continued until the ulcer was clean and healing, with no growth from swab cultures. A further 2 months of regular dressings of the ulcer by the practice nurse and fortnightly review at the diabetes centre resulted in a healed ulcer and excellent diabetic control (HbA_{1C}, 6.5%). Follow-up was arranged at the general practice surgery. Avoiding injuries in future was discussed and the patient was warned to attend promptly if there were any further problems.

Infection in a diabetic patient increases insulin resistance and leads to poor glycaemic control. Poor control delays healing and the increasing spiral of worsening control and spreading infection is dangerous. In this situation, tight glycaemic control (blood glucose 4–7 mmol/l and HbA_{1C} in the normal range) is essential and aggressive antibiotic therapy is imperative.

Case 5: Patient concerns about hypoglycaemia unawareness

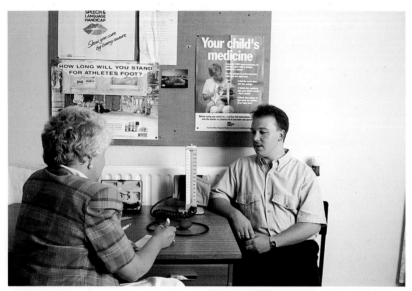

Reproduced with permission from Bubbles/H.C. Robinson

A 25-year-old man with insulin dependent diabetes mellitus (IDDM) for 20 years tells his family practitioner that the previous day he had a driving accident while hypoglycaemic. He has been warned by the police to stop driving, but he needs to drive for his job as a car mechanic. He has had problems with hypoglycaemic attacks and has lost the warning symptoms of hypoglycaemia. He is convinced that human insulin is the cause and wishes to change back to animal insulin.

Family practitioner. To ease the patient's worries, a change to porcine insulin was agreed. His insulin regimen consisted of fast-acting plus intermediate-acting insulins twice daily. As his hypoglycaemic episodes have been occurring in the evening, a reduction in the evening fast-acting insulin dose was proposed.

Original insulin	a.m.	p.m.	New insulin	a.m.	p.m.
Actrapid	20	18	Velosulin porcine	20	16
Monotard	30	26	Insulatard porcine	30	26

The patient agreed to see the diabetologist for further advice.

Diabetologist. A few weeks later, hypoglycaemic attacks were still a problem, so a complete reappraisal was required. Arrangements were made for the patient to see the dietitian and the diabetes nurse specialist.

For someone with a job involving considerable physical activity, he was taking quite large doses of fast-acting insulin. In an attempt to avoid hypoglycaemia, which was now a problem both mid-morning and evening, his fast-acting insulin doses were reduced still further.

Dietitian. This patient's carbohydrate intake varied considerably from day to day. He did not consistently eat between-meal snacks and his meals tended to consist of fast foods, such as pasties or fish and chips. He was advised to eat more bread, cereals and potatoes at mealtimes and not to fill up with fatty foods.

Diabetes nurse specialist. The patient was depressed and frightened by severe hypoglycaemic episodes and the car accident. It became clear that he was adjusting his food intake according to home blood glucose monitoring results. The last severe hypoglycaemic attack was prompted by a blood glucose result of 12 mmol/l at lunch time and his response of eating only half his lunch. He agreed to try and stabilize his food intake.

Together, we attempted to avoid hypoglycaemia and indeed any readings of less than 4 mmol/l, by further adjustment of his insulin doses, but were unsuccessful.

Diabetologist. A trial period of multiple injection therapy (MIT) was agreed and the patient was commenced on 10 units of Velosulin before breakfast, lunch and the evening meal and 24 units of Insulatard at bedtime. It is always difficult to judge the correct doses when switching to MIT. Generally, total insulin requirements are lower and a significant reduction with a later adjustment, if necessary, is a wise step.

Diabetes nurse specialist. After high initial blood glucose results, doses were increased until the patient finally stabilized on 12, 12 and 16 units of Velosulin and 30 units of Insulatard. For the convenience of an insulin pen, he was willing to return to human insulin, Actrapid and Insulatard, as he now accepts that it had played no part in his problems.

Diabetologist. After 4 months of MIT, the patient has reasonable control (HbA$_{1c}$, 7.5%) and has regained his confidence. He has had no severe hypoglycaemic attacks for 3 months and has regained his warning symptoms. He will apply to the driving authorities and with my medical report emphasizing these points will probably be granted a licence. A follow-up plan has been agreed with his family practitioner and the diabetes nurse specialist.

Patients can regain their warning symptoms of hypoglycaemia by careful adjustment of their diabetes management, regular snacks and meals, and frequent monitoring of blood glucose levels (see pages 112–14). Clearly, all this requires hard work and commitment.

Case 6: Painful neuropathy

A woman who was 56 years old and with NIDDM diagnosed only 3 months previously, presented with a severe burning pain on the left side of her chest, which had caused sleepless nights for 2 weeks. Simple analgesics did not help.

Family practitioner. Her diabetes was coming under control with diet alone.

Results

	Plasma glucose (mmol/l)	HbA$_{1C}$(%)*	Weight (kg)
At diagnosis	15.5 (2-hour post-meal)	10.3	74
Diet (3 months)	7.0 (fasting)	7.5	71
Diet (4.5 months)	7.8 (fasting)	8.0	68
Diet (7 months) + gliclazide, 40mg/day	6.1 (fasting)	5.9	70

*Normal range = 4.1–6.5%

Examination did not disclose a cause for the pain and stronger analgesics (codeine plus paracetamol) were prescribed. Two weeks later, the patient returned with no improvement. The differential diagnosis of shingles was unlikely as lesions were absent and the time course did not fit. Regular dihydrocodeine was prescribed and the patient was referred to the hospital diabetes clinic.

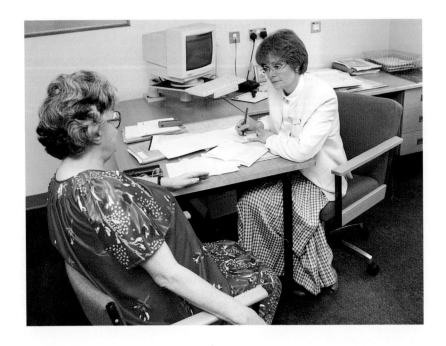

Diabetologist. A few weeks following referral, the patient's condition had worsened. She could bear only very loose clothing and described a pain like an electric shock whenever clothing touched her skin on the left side of her chest or abdomen. An area of marked hyperaesthesia was apparent on examination. It was confined to the left side of the body but fitted no clear dermatome pattern. There were no skin changes and no other neurological abnormality.

The patient had an acute painful diabetic neuropathy or 'neuritis'. Although uncommon, most diabetologists see one or two cases a year. It is most likely that this case resulted from the fall in blood glucose levels after diagnosis following years of unrecognized hyperglycaemia. The hyperaesthesia is probably associated with damaged nerves undergoing regeneration. Unlike certain other forms of neuropathy, this condition is transient, though recovery may take 3–18 months. The patient was relieved to receive an explanation for the pain.

Treatment of any painful diabetic neuropathy is difficult. The maintenance of excellent glycaemic control will hasten recovery, and this should be stressed to the patient. Recent assessment showed some deterioration in the patient's glycaemic control. Gliclazide, 80 mg/day, was introduced but hypoglycaemic episodes prompted a dose reduction to 40 mg/day, when control became excellent.

Physical treatments may be helpful. For example, wearing a close-fitting garment prevents pain arising from outer garments brushing against the skin. A transcutaneous electrical nerve stimulator can sometimes be useful.

Carbamazepine or amitryptyline may be valuable as they may raise the pain threshold and therefore help sleep. Their role should be explained carefully to the patient or expectations will not be met. This patient responded well to amitryptyline after increasing the dose gradually from 50 mg to 100 mg nocte. After 10 months, the pain disappeared, but during this time the patient required constant support and reassurance.

Case 7: Foot ulcer

A 30-year-old diabetic patient presented to his family practitioner with a painful swollen foot. He had had insulin-dependent diabetes (IDDM) for 20 years and was treated with twice-daily Humulin S plus Humulin I.

Family practitioner. This patient had been an erratic attender for diabetic reviews in the past. When I examined his foot, I was concerned because it was red, hot and swollen, with a spreading cellulitis from an ulcer on the sole. On closer questioning, the patient admitted trying to remove some hard skin on the sole of his foot. Cephradine, 500 mg q.d.s., was prescribed, as he was allergic to penicillin, and arrangements were made for the practice nurse to swab and dress the ulcer. An urgent appointment was arranged at the hospital diabetic clinic.

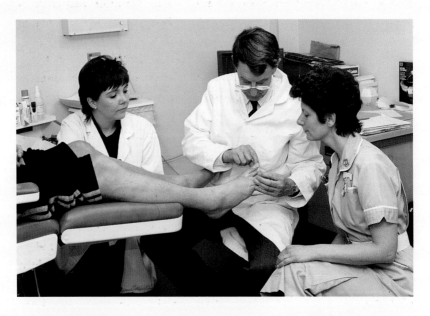

A team approach to diabetic foot disease, involving the chiropodist, diabetologist and nurse, is essential.

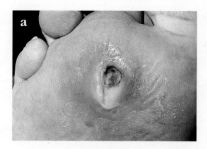 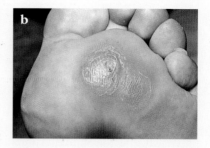

Following treatment to improve the cellulitis and remove some callus; **a** *1-cm ulcer in area of high pressure under the second metatarsal head;* **b** *left foot: no ulcer, but callus developing in area of high pressure under the second metatarsal head.*

Diabetologist. The patient attended the diabetic foot clinic the following day. There were signs of peripheral neuropathy, with impaired light touch and vibration sense in both feet, ankle reflexes were absent and there was callus on the plantar surface of both feet, with a 1-cm diameter ulcer on the right foot. The ulcer was emitting pus and there was surrounding cellulitis. The gravity of the situation prompted immediate admission to hospital.

At the suggestion of his family practitioner, the patient had started monitoring his blood glucose, and reported levels of 15–20 mmol/l. The HbA$_{1C}$ result was 9.5% (normal range, 4.1–6.5%). The infection was leading to deteriorating glycaemic control, which would result in delayed healing and escalating infection. Spreading infection can destroy the tissues and necessitate amputation.

In hospital, antibiotics were given intravenously, and diabetes was brought under control by switching to multiple injection therapy (Humulin S before each meal and Humulin I at bedtime). The insulin doses were increased until all blood glucose results were from 4–7 mmol/l. In this situation, excellent glycaemic control is imperative.

A radiograph of the foot showed no evidence of osteomyelitis. Debridement of the callus was undertaken by the chiropodist and strict bed rest was ordered. Fortunately, the infection resolved quickly and with weekly chiropody, appropriate footwear and regular dressing, the ulcer healed in 2 months.

Chiropodist. This ulcer, infection and hospital admission were preventable. The patient was at high risk of ulcer development because of neuropathy and high-pressure areas under his feet. He needed to attend an ulcer prevention programme for education on how to avoid these problems (see page 218). In the long term, regular chiropody to remove the excessive callus and insoles in the shoes to reduce high pressure under the second metatarsal head should prevent further ulceration. The annual review examination, which this patient failed to attend, needs to identify such patients and institute preventive measures.

Case 8: Conversion to insulin treatment

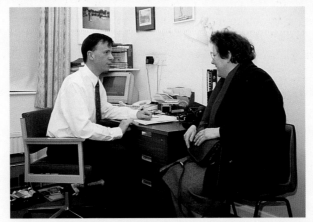

Reproduced with permission from Dr P. Marazzi/ Science Photo Library.

An overweight 62-year-old woman, who had had non-insulin dependent diabetes mellitus (NIDDM) for 10 years, presents to her family practitioner for review.

CLINICAL RECORD

Date	Plasma Glucose	HbA₁c	Weight	BMI (Kg/m²)	Treatment
2·2·95	8·9	9·2	75kg	32	Chlorpropamide, 15mg os
2·8·95	9·3	8·9	74·5kg	32	+ Metformin, 850mg bd
4·1·96	9·5	10·5	75kg	32	
14·6·96	8·1	10·2	74kg	32	
13·12·96	9·9	10·8	74kg	32	

The patient's co-operation book illustrates her suboptimal glycaemic control over the past 2 years.

Family practitioner. This patient's glycaemic control has been definitely suboptimal (HbA$_{1c}$, 8–10%; normal range, 4.1–6.5%) for several years though she takes glibenclamide, 15 mg/day, and metformin, 850 mg b.d. Both higher doses of metformin and a trial of low-dose acarbose have led to diarrhoea. I am reluctant to consider insulin as she is so overweight (body mass index, 32 kg/m^2), though her weight is constant and she does her best to follow her diet. She reports no symptoms and has no complications.

Diabetologist. This patient presents a common dilemma: poor glycaemic control with persistent obesity. The options are to:
- maintain on maximal oral hypoglycaemic agents
- convert to insulin treatment.

Deteriorating glycaemic control with time is the natural history of NIDDM whatever the form of treatment (see page 88).

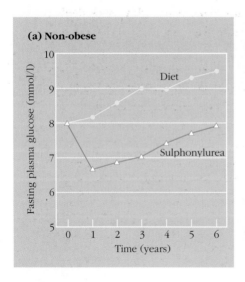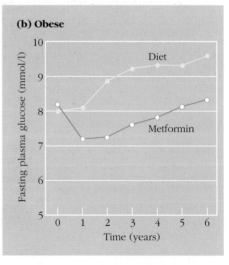

Deteriorating glycaemic control is the natural history of NIDDM, as shown here by results from the UK Prospective Diabetes Study[1].

Poor glycaemic control is associated with increased risk of microvascular complications and therefore, the first step is to review the patient and check that her dietary compliance seems reasonable. The next step I would recommend is a 6-month trial of insulin treatment to assess whether she will tolerate it and whether her glycaemic control improves. The proposed insulin regimen is twice-daily premixed insulins given by insulin pen (e.g. Mixtard 30® or Humaject M3®). Although glibenclamide is to be withdrawn, metformin should be continued. Using insulin plus metformin improves insulin sensitivity and may restrict the weight gain that often results from insulin treatment.

If the patient is not commenced on insulin, worsening glycaemic control and the development of complications would be likely consequences. In my opinion, initiating insulin treatment is often delayed unnecessarily. The majority of patients report that they feel better with insulin treatment even if they had no symptoms previously. Glycaemic control often takes 6 months to settle and HbA_{1c} should fall to 7–8%. Weight gain should be restricted to less than 2 kg with metformin in the regimen.

Although the practice of 'evidence based medicine' is desirable, there is as yet no evidence to guide physicians in this situation. In the future, results of the UK Prospective Diabetes Study may prove helpful.

Reference

1 UK Prospective Diabetes Study Group. U.K. Prospective Diabetes Study 16. Overview of 6 years' therapy of type II diabetes: a progressive disease. *Diabetes* 1995; **44:** 1249–58.

Index